Stroke – It Couldn't Happen to Me

ONE WOMAN'S STORY OF SURVIVING
A BRAIN-STEM STROKE

Stroke – It Couldn't Happen to Me

ONE WOMAN'S STORY OF SURVIVING A BRAIN-STEM STROKE

MARGARET CROMARTY

Foreword by
DERICK WADE
Consultant and Professor in Neurological
Rehabilitation, Oxford

Radcliffe Publishing
Oxford • New York

Radcliffe Publishing Ltd
18 Marcham Road
Abingdon
Oxon OX14 1AA
United Kingdom

www.radcliffe-oxford.com
Electronic catalogue and worldwide online ordering facility.

British Library Cataloguing in Publication Data

A catalogue record for this book is available from the British Library.

ISBN-13: 978 1 84619 295 1

Typeset by Pindar New Zealand (Egan Reid), Auckland, New Zealand
Printed and bound by TJI Digital, Padstow, Cornwall, UK

Contents

To my fantastic family.

Foreword

I remember vividly my first meeting with Margaret. She was lying in an intensive care unit surrounded by very ill people. She, like them, was attached to various monitors and tubes all bleeping, and dripping and draining fluids. But she was obviously awake, and extremely keen to communicate. And, although it was then slow and laborious, communicate she did.

I also recall the day for another reason. After leaving her, I travelled with my specialist registrar to London to see another patient, a man a few years older also in an intensive care unit after acute brain damage. He was totally unresponsive, and in the vegetative state. Until that point my registrar had wondered how one could distinguish the 'locked-in state' from the 'vegetative state'. The vibrant life in Margaret contrasted with its complete absence in my second patient. My registrar was never concerned about making the distinction again.

Margaret has influenced and improved all who have known her. She tolerated her wait to be transferred to Rivermead Rehabilitation Centre without complaint (and she could certainly complain if she wanted to). She helped us learn about her condition and what it meant to be in such a state. She had unshakable faith, and at no time did she seem to doubt that she would succeed in getting home. That determination and certainty helped everyone who was helping her; many of the staff had not seen anyone so dependent before and did not believe it was possible for someone in her state to get home.

Of course Margaret was not alone. She was supported throughout by her husband and children, and conversely she worked hard so that she could continue to be an active part of their lives. And she has, as you will read.

Finally, Margaret has steadfastly kept in touch with me, which is unusual and helps us put ourselves in context. Specialist rehabilitation centres such as Rivermead may consider themselves important. However, for the person who has experienced a sudden onset severely disabling condition, their involvement with rehabilitation is only a phase. The time people spend at specialist centres such as Rivermead is just a short time, as school is for most people. Hopefully, it helps the person learn how to live, but it cannot make them live a full life. Margaret has repaid many times over the efforts we made.

Margaret has gone on to live a full life, albeit different from that anticipated. Read this and be interested, but do not feel sad, or distressed, or pity. Margaret is very much alive, very much an equal part of her family and community, and is arguably a more important and influential member of Society than she used to be.

Derick Wade
Consultant and Professor in
Neurological Rehabilitation, Oxford
July 2008

About the author

Margaret Cromarty SRN(Retired), DipHSW(Open) was 43 when she had a massive stroke in 1999. 'Locked-in' for four months, she could only communicate by blinking. Gradual improvements still left her quadraplegic and barely able to talk, but with the efforts of her family she was able to go home and lead a relatively normal life. An ex-nurse and RAF wife, she is married with two grown-up daughters.

During the first year after Margaret's stroke, her husband, Iain, kept a journal – this can be viewed online at www.radcliffe-oxford.com/patientnarratives.

1. The day the sky fell in

It was Mothering Sunday. Our younger daughter, Elisabeth, was away at boarding school. We had no plans to see her that weekend because she would soon be home for the holiday. Our elder daughter, Elinor, was fast asleep after a late night out with friends. My mother was staying with us; I had collected her from the station the day before.

The three of us sat down for breakfast. Mum and I planned to go to church; Iain, being an atheist, wouldn't go so he was going to write his first essay for the Open University. On the table was a beautiful bunch of anemones, the tissue paper they were wrapped in matched the blue flowers and set off the red. I was entranced. Obviously Elisabeth had dispatched Elinor to buy them on her behalf. I gave Mum her present: a scarf and a big box of chocolates.

After breakfast Mum and I set off for church, while Iain went up to the computer. It was a lovely day. I didn't have to prepare lunch as after church we were all going to my sister's. The service was a joint one with the church down the road but was held at ours.

We chatted for a while with our friends and then it was time for the service to begin. The children were called to the front to collect a plant for each mother and then for all the other ladies in the church. Last year Elinor and Elisabeth qualified as ladies much to their delight, each receiving a pretty plant from the children. This time, after the children had each taken their mothers a flower, Mum and I both received a lovely big primula. We all settled down to listen to the sermon.

A few minutes later the world began to spin. I was quite alarmed but it soon subsided and all seemed well. Then I began to feel dizzy again and I felt peculiar down my left side. The noise in my head distorted the wise words of the minister and I felt distinctly abnormal.

"There is something wrong with me" I hissed at my mother, while trying to sit perfectly still.

"Do you want to go out?" she asked but I replied that I didn't dare move. I was afraid that I would fall to the left. I continued to sit very still and I kept my eyes tightly closed because the world was still jumping.

After a while, which on reflection can only have been half a minute, I became aware that my friend, who sits on the other side of the church, had come over and put her arm round me. She too asked if I wanted to go out but my mum told her that I dare not move. Meanwhile the sermon continued, but I was oblivious to it and to everything beyond my efforts not to fall over and not to be noticed. In the end, after some discussion, my mum, my friend and another friend who was sitting behind us took me by the arms and frogmarched me out to the entrance hall.

Once there we were joined by another friend who is a nurse and she, businesslike, took control of the situation. I made to sit down on one of the chairs but I was persuaded to lie along four pushed together.

"I think I am having a stroke," I quipped, recognising the symptoms and thinking it was mildly amusing given my age – just 43 – and never suspecting it could result in anything more serious than some slight one-sided weakness for a while.

"Oh no," was the horrified response from the nurse, "it could be lots of other things." I had my doubts and suggested that they fetch Iain, my GP husband. My friend phoned him from the minister's office and I lay still with my eyes closed.

Moments later Iain arrived and my friends told him the sequence of events.

"Have I got **nystagmus?**" I asked, still feeling objective about the whole business. The characteristic flickering of my eyes would explain why the world was jumping. Iain confirmed that I had, and quickly ran through all my symptoms.

"I think we had better go to casualty," said Iain – I could sense the gravity of the situation from his demeanour. I did not argue. I was helped to the car and we drove off, thinking this was rather inconvenient. We had so many plans, not only for that day but also for the weeks ahead.

It did not take long to drive to the local district general

hospital. We parked illegally in the ambulance bay and Iain ran in to prepare the staff for my arrival. Minutes later a man in uniform, presumably a porter, came out to the car with a wheelchair.

"How do you feel?" he said, to which I replied, "peculiar". For peculiar it was, not unlike being horribly drunk with a left-sided list.

I was wheeled into a small room and a nurse came to see me. For the first time I heard the word **CVA** (which I knew to be the posh word for stroke) as the porter handed over my notes. Still I remained vaguely amused and objective about it all, discussing the goings on with my husband and even making philosophical observations about my predicament. However the large painted cartoon figures on the wall continued to do gymnastics every time I opened my eyes.

Time passed. All sorts of examinations were carried out, and an **IV infusion** was put up 'just in case'. I chatted on to the nurses, doctors and Iain. After a while my speech became slurred.

"I am going off," I observed. Although I was still feeling objective, I began to feel that this was serious, perhaps worth more than the amused consideration I had previously given it. We discussed ways of communicating if I became unintelligible. We decided on one blink for yes and two for no. That was to prove my salvation in the weeks to come.

Sometime during the afternoon I was given a brain scan; we were delighted to be told that I didn't have a tumour or a haemorrhage – there was no mention of the clot which was the actual cause of the whole business.

Iain was beginning to make noises about sending for Elisabeth; despatching someone to fetch her back from school. He telephoned home to let Elinor and my mother know what was going on. At least I didn't need to worry about them; my sister was bringing lunch to our house, so they would be all together and catered for, so to speak.

During the afternoon I was visited and examined by several doctors, the most notable of whom was the medical registrar. He sat down and explained how the brain is like a cauliflower, with the brain stem as the stalk. I had a clot where the stalk joins the rest of the cauliflower. This could have serious consequences.

"Will I die?" I asked, never expecting an answer in the affirmative. After a pause the doctor replied, "I must be perfectly honest; it is possible. We must wait for the stroke to evolve". Evolve? I had no idea that strokes evolved. I thought that the damage was done and that was that. For the first time I became really worried. I might die. Inside I felt great turmoil. Outwardly I tried to be calm and matter-of-fact. Iain and I discussed the future in the event of my death. Elinor was to go to university and pursue her planned career, and Elisabeth must go ahead and sit her GCSEs, due in the summer. As for Iain, I wished that I could find it in my heart to give my blessing to him finding someone else. However, I have always been a possessive creature and even under these circumstances couldn't bear the thought of him with another woman – so drew the line at that. Life insurance would provide the means to buy a family home when Iain left the Royal Air Force at the end of the year.

When he next suggested sending for Elisabeth I acquiesced (with a sense of foreboding) so Iain's brother was despatched to collect her. A little later Elinor, my mother and my sister came in to see what was going on and found me leaning to the left, my speech deteriorating markedly. I began to communicate by pointing at letters written out large, spelling the words I wanted to say.

Meanwhile, a bed had to be found for me somewhere in the hospital. It was decided that I shouldn't go to the emergency admissions ward, as Elinor frequently worked there as an **HCA**, and it was deemed inappropriate that I should be one of her patients. I was sent to the female medical ward which was inhabited, it seemed, by elderly long-stay patients. It seemed that the staff didn't know how to deal with emergencies; they were certainly ill-equipped to do so. As my condition deteriorated, or "went off" as I described it at the time, there was a lack of basic resuscitation equipment and/or the knowledge of how or when to use it. I learned later that Iain was afraid that night that I might die, not from the stroke itself, but 'by accident' because of the absence of adequate care on the ward

During the night, it became necessary to give me a **urinary catheter** because my bladder wasn't working properly and, with Iain keeping vigil by my bedside, I got worse. By morning I was completely paralysed and unable to speak.

2. Locked-in

It is the stuff of nightmares. How often have we, as children, come out in a sweat imagining being unable to move? But this was no figment of the imagination. The only part of me which could move was my left eyelid. My eyes would move up and down but not side to side. But I was well aware of what was going on. At first there was no time to dwell on things because of the rushing around that went on.

There was a big flap because I was not breathing properly. On the way to the ambulance which was to take me to the Regional Centre I was intubated. The family came to say goodbye (not knowing if it was to be forever) and I was anaesthetised before setting off in the ambulance to the bigger hospital.

I don't know how long it took, but I came to in the Intensive Care Unit. The rest of that day is very hazy. I was a mass of tubes and wires. There was a **nasogastric tube**, through which I was to be fed, and a long line into my groin, through which an **angiogram** had been performed, to look at the blood vessels supplying my brain. There was also an **arterial line** in my left wrist. Of course there was also the urinary catheter as well.

Over the next few days I lost count of the number of needles I had stuck in me. There were blood tests done, intravenous infusions resited, and after a day or two, a **tracheostomy** performed so that the **endotracheal tube** could be removed from my mouth and oxygen be passed straight from the ventilator into my airway.

This was done under anaesthetic, which was just as well because I wouldn't have liked to have been awake for that. I might have seemed brave, putting up with all the things that were done to me, but really I had no choice. I couldn't shout and I couldn't flinch; I had to suffer in silence.

The episode with the tracheostomy is a good example of my experience while 'locked-in'. I understood everything that was said. I still had opinions. I still had standards. I had fears, questions, humour, impatience. In short, I thought just as I had always done. Iain had established early on that I was 'in there somewhere' so we had 'discussed' the pros and cons of having a tracheostomy. The doctor, however, assumed that I was incapable of understanding or giving consent to the operation, so he asked Iain to give his on my behalf. This annoyed both of us. Iain became my advocate, pointing out to all comers that I was intelligent and should be treated as such, even though there would be no response from me.

We worked on our 'code', developing it from the eye-blink to an up/down flash of the eyes. In this way I was able to 'converse' with members of my family. Iain and his brother both made notices to put above my bed. One had two recent photographs of me, with the caption 'Please remember – this is me'; the other one was a list of things I could and couldn't do, such as 'I can hear and understand, and I cannot move or speak'. I didn't feel quite as much panic as I might have done as I knew that Iain and the girls believed that I was still 'with it' and treated me accordingly. I did however feel dreadful despair, thinking of the things that I did so easily and oh so recently. They seemed to have gone forever. People who didn't know me tended to treat me as though the stroke had affected me mentally. I longed to put them straight with some sharp remark but, of course, I was doomed to lie silent. The nurses were very good, always addressing me as Mrs Cromarty and speaking to me as an intelligent human being but ancillary staff, such as radiographers and part-time physiotherapists, were condescending or patronising, which used to infuriate me. Perhaps the most upsetting was the attitude of the senior doctors. Was it my imagination that they shot me sympathetic glances, and muttered "tsk tsk" as they hurried past? I felt written-off. On the scrapheap at forty three.

The despair I felt knew no bounds. I had never heard of 'Locked-In Syndrome'. But I began to hear the term used in reference to me. My mind, as quick and as 'healthy' as it ever had been, was 'locked-in' my useless body. There was no way out. I couldn't talk, nor make a noise of any sort. I couldn't nod or shake my head, nor gesticulate in any way. I was completely passive. If anyone said "hello", I could only stare. It was very much against the grain but whenever anything was done for me I couldn't say "thank you". Neither could I shout out in pain if something hurt. I just lay like an inert lump and thought my thoughts. I became totally reliant on the nurses needing to carry out their routine tasks with me to secure their company, as I could not call for help. This was not too much of a problem in **ITU**, as each patient was allocated a nurse in constant attendance, but I felt particularly vulnerable as I moved on to the **High Dependency Unit** and later to the main ward. I would worry from visit to visit, afraid that something might happen and I wouldn't be able to attract attention. While on the ward I used to have quite violent coughing fits, which propelled me to the edge of the bed. I would often lie in this precarious position, unable to call out, until a passer-by noticed me, when something would eventually be done.

I have been told that when I was locked-in, lying motionless and expressionless, my face was perfectly smooth. Not a line or wrinkle in sight. Smooth it might have been, but also completely characterless. My daughters have told me since that it was more through faith than certainty that they believed that I was still 'with it'. Meanwhile my mind was racing, as it normally did. I reminded myself of a patient I nursed some years ago. I, to my shame, assumed like everyone else that because she couldn't move, had frequent spasms of her limbs, and didn't speak, she didn't know what was going on and was completely devoid of thought and feeling. The curtains were always drawn around her bed and she received the minimum necessary nursing care. She was somewhat of an embarrassment on our busy surgical ward. With horror I realised that she could well have known exactly what was going on, for wasn't I in a similar position? I was perfectly aware of everything even though I lay seemingly lifelessly. When a **gastrostomy** was suggested, to put liquid food straight into my stomach, the similarity seemed complete. Despair hung over me as I imagined ending up hidden away somewhere, considered mentally 'dead' by everyone. Thankfully my family and friends had other ideas.

Iain devised a way for us to communicate. He would run through the alphabet and I would blink on the appropriate letter as he came to it, so that I could build up words that I wanted to say. So we could 'converse', albeit slowly, and thus I began to feel less isolated. I felt reasonably confident when Iain was around, and very soon also when I was with the girls. I felt that, rather than regarding me as some 'thing', they would take the time to find the person I had always been, still there in that useless body.

Perhaps the worst thing about my predicament was the fact that I had no control over anything. The most basic things had to be done or aided by something or someone else. Firstly my breathing was helped by a ventilator. Although I initiated each breath, the machine took over, ensuring that a proper breath was taken each time. Within a few days the aforementioned tracheostomy was performed to allow the endotracheal tube to be removed from my mouth. Feeding was taken care of through the nasogastric tube and weeks later by the gastrostomy. Waterworks were dealt with by the catheter. I needed to be turned regularly from side to side to keep my skin free from the effects of pressure. Basic nursing care such as washing and cleaning my mouth and teeth were of course necessary. In addition, I depended on others (usually nurses) to do things for me that I would never have dreamt of asking anyone else to do before, such as removing a stray hair from my eye, shaving my armpits, or changing my sanitary pad during periods. The first time that my husband cleaned inside my nose with a cotton-bud I was mortified, but as he explained, he knew I would hate to be seen with a runny nose, and of course he was right. He continued to do similar things for me. Often I would lie and hope that someone would notice that I needed something, or that someone would read my mind. It was dreadful not to be able to scratch my face or rub my eyes. I had great cause to be thankful for the many years of yoga I'd done. I had learned some breathing and relaxation techniques over time which proved immensely helpful when I was having something unpleasant done to me or when I was tempted to fight the paralysis that had taken over my body. I entertained the notion that there was an element of 'mind over matter' involved, and that if I tried hard enough I would be able to make things work. Of course that wasn't the case at all, and I very soon learned that there was little point in struggling against the impossible and I consciously relaxed rather than fought to no avail.

Most of my waking time was spent watching the comings and goings around me. Both in ITU and in the **High Dependency Unit (HDU)** I could see the nurses' station, where the nurses would congregate and where I could observe shift changes. I also watched the doorway into the unit through which my family would appear: an event I eagerly awaited each day. Of course I could not greet them properly; a blink of the eye had to suffice, and that only with my left as the right would not shut properly. During those early days only close family members and close friends came to see me. I was glad of that as I didn't want to be seen in that condition – I wouldn't look in a mirror, vain that I was even then. One medical visitor I had was the director of the local rehabilitation centre, which is fortuitously among the leading centres in the country for the rehabilitation of head injury and stroke victims. He spent some time with members of my family, explaining the possible and even likely outcomes of my situation (severe disablement and only partial speech). These were relayed back to me, supposedly to give me encouragement, but I was unimpressed. Nothing short of complete recovery, with a return to how I was before the stroke, would do. No matter that I had 'Locked-In Syndrome', a rare state in which a person suffers a collection of almost insurmountable problems following a brain stem stroke, resulting in a perfectly alert mind being trapped in an absolutely useless body.

I was promised a place in the rehabilitation centre sometime in the future. Meanwhile the director suggested that when we were spelling out words we divide the alphabet into two, from A to M and from N to Z. Every letter was preceded by the question, "Is it in the first or the second half of the alphabet?"

I would reply by looking upwards for the first half and downwards for the second. This saved time and although this system was still slow, we were able to have quite fluent conversations. Every visitor was tutored in this code by Iain and the brave among them made a reasonable attempt at talking with me. We carried on with this for several months; it made my locked-in state less unbearable – at least while the family was around.

I continued to be 'locked-in' throughout my days in ITU

and during my time in the HDU. After a couple of weeks I was transferred to the general neurological ward. I continued to be visited by the same senior doctor. One day I was following his finger with my eyes (a regularly-performed neurological test) when I kept following the finger, turning my head to keep it in view. This was the first time I had moved anything. I was quite excited; the nurse in attendance was moved to tears.

On another occasion, within days of this, I was visited by a particularly irritating member of staff. After he had left, I started to spell out a word to my assembled family, C – R – E . . .

"Creep," interjected my sister, a bit doubtful whether that was the word that was coming. Everyone laughed, and I joined in. For the first time I broke into a grin, albeit a lopsided one (at this stage only the left side of my face showed any sign of life.)

I was beginning to Break Out . . .

3. Live or let die

The first few days after the stroke were hellish, for me and for my loved ones. My departure from the local hospital was alarming for us all. I remember a high-speed dash on a trolley along the myriad corridors; my family remembers bidding farewell before the journey to the bigger hospital, not knowing whether or not it was for the last time. There was some talk of a risky procedure to try to dissolve the clot. It might not even work. I decided to go ahead with it; after all I wanted to get back to normal as soon as possible. We had so many plans for the days and weeks ahead. As it happened, the procedure failed, there was no instant improvement, and an angiogram of my neck and head showed not only the clot but also the bad state of some of the vessels supplying my brain. It seemed that I was doomed.

Of course I knew very little of this. When I was in ITU I was attached to a ventilator. There was a big fat tube (the endotracheal tube, connecting my lungs to the ventilator) in my mouth. I lay motionless on my back, and people talked at me in calm and soothing tones. I felt completely bewildered. Although I did not know it at the time, the ventilator was set to help me breathe after I had initiated each breath. It was up to me to keep breathing. It was hard work. I felt dreadful. There was a loud ringing in my ears, I couldn't move, and I felt hellishly uncomfortable. Although I couldn't move, I could feel everything; I felt discomfort and pain just as I always had. Fortunately, I didn't have any pain unless anyone did something unpleasant to me.

So I just lay there breathing, listening, watching and thinking. What a mess! I could not see a way out of this. What sort of life was this anyway? And it was so hard to breathe. I was no use to anyone in this condition. Least of all to myself. It looked as though the best thing for all concerned would be for me to let go. After all, think of the life insurance. Iain and the girls would be able to buy the sort of home we had always planned, and there might be no need for a mortgage.

But wait a minute! I was not ready for eternal oblivion! I had long held the opinion that death was preferable to a poor quality of life, but now that it was my life at stake I felt very differently. I might miss something! Our daughters would soon embark on their chosen careers, might settle down with husbands and have children – my grandchildren – and I wanted to be around. Besides, I had waited years for Iain and me to have our own home, out of the RAF, and we were nearly there. Was I going to let that go? What about the prospect of Iain and a new wife? No Way! I made up my mind to fight. I did not want to die. But it was so difficult to breathe. It felt as though there was a heavy weight on my chest, trying to prevent me from inhaling. Every breath was a supreme effort. All I could think about was taking the next breath in. One breath after another. I don't remember for how many hours or days this went on. I do remember two occasions when I was terrified that I would die; each breath was incredibly hard. Somehow I kept going.

One time, my mother was sitting with me. She leaned forward and, adopting her best schoolmarm voice, urged: "Don't you DARE give up on us". I thought ruefully that I was doing my best, but wasn't sure that it would be good enough. I recalled that tone, albeit fiercer and less choked than this, from my childhood. Then I would certainly have done as I was told on hearing it. But this time I recognised that it was more of a plea than an admonition. So I fought for my life, and somehow managed to survive that initial hurdle.

I learned later that the doctors expected that I would die. They made a poor attempt at concealing this expectation. They discussed me over me. I was dismayed at the negative vibes they exuded each time they came to see me. I felt that they had written me off already. Of course they can have had little idea of how their behaviour affected me. I just lay there, seemingly unresponsive, just existing, unable to enlighten them as to what was going on inside my head. Days passed, one monotonously after another, and I did not die. Although I was given good care, and nothing I needed was withheld, nothing heroic was done to keep me alive. I felt that I was on my own, left to sink or swim. Of course I was not alone; my family and friends were, and still are, right behind me. But I felt that the medical staff had abandoned me to my fate. *Right*, I thought belligerently, when feeling a little less scared, *I'll show them*! And I determined to work as hard as it took to get back to normal.

4. Reality and unreality

I still have difficulty believing that this situation is real. After all, this sort of thing doesn't happen to me. Does it? Why not? Why should I be any different from anyone else? Many people encounter tragedy in some form or other during the course of their lives. Did I think that I was immune? Well, yes. I did. My life had been relatively straightforward so far. The only really traumatic time I can readily identify was when my father died suddenly, just over eight years before. I was distraught, grieving for over a year and needing counselling to help me get through the early months.

Until now, my life had followed a reasonable path. I had had a secure and happy childhood, brought up in a close family in a small rural town, where everyone knew everyone else, and, in some cases, everyone else's business too. A little precocious I fear, I excelled at music, was 'big' in Girl Guiding, and was Head Girl at primary school. I was a bossy child (perhaps my talent for organisation originated here), and must have given my younger sister a pretty rough time. A 'big fish in a small pond', I soon became a 'small fish in a big pond' when I went to the local grammar school. This took some adjustment but it was probably what I needed. In my class was a boy named Iain, who was to become my husband, but whom I had very little to do with until the end of the sixth form. I left school with eight 'O' levels and three 'A' levels, and set off for London to do my nursing training. Iain went to Edinburgh to study medicine, and as we had just got together, there began three years of daily letter writing. At the end of the three years it took for me to get my nursing registration, we got married and I went to join Iain in Edinburgh.

We spent two and a half happy years there. I worked as a staff nurse on a surgical ward and then in a busy casualty department during this time while Iain finished his studies and did his year as a houseman. After this time we had to go where the RAF sent us. It was payback time.

Iain had received a salary from the Air Force while he was at university and now, in return, he had to serve at least five years. At least! Our five years turned into twenty and became a bone of contention between us for a long time. We moved to Cornwall, I gave up earning a living, and we decided to start a family. Making babies was for us as easy as falling off a log, and our elder daughter was born less than a year later. Giving birth, however, was nowhere near as easy, and a Caesarean section was required to produce not only our elder daughter but also our younger, just over two years afterwards. Elinor, our elder, was a happy baby although the pregnancy and time around her birth were a misery to me. Elisabeth, however, was a very crabby baby, getting me up every night until she was two years old. I had been much happier during this pregnancy than the last, and the time surrounding Elisabeth's birth had been much more pleasant. Perhaps I was getting to be an 'old hand'! By the time our family was complete we were on our fourth home, courtesy of the RAF, and we would go on to have ten more before we were able to leave and settle down in our own place. I tended to blame any rough patches in our marriage upon the various aspects of our life in the services, whether or not this was fair. It was not without its difficulties. Not least of these were the frequent moves. I never liked packing my treasures and all our possessions into an assortment of cardboard boxes – I always worried that I might never see them again, or that they would end up in pieces. The need to make new friends, find one's way around a different shopping centre, register with a new dentist and so on, was at best tedious and at its worst a dreadful headache. I did get used to the packing up and even got slick at it but I always loathed the moving.

Another bone of contention was the drinking. Life in the services seems to be synonymous with alcohol. Not that I found that in itself a problem; I am very fond of a drink or two myself. But I despise drunkenness, and I would lose patience with the apparent need (or expectation) to 'get drunk with the boys in the bar'. There seemed to be some magical camaraderie involved in this, but it was beyond me and I was frequently very vociferous with my objections.

Despite this disapproval of our lifestyle, I still made, according to Iain, an excellent RAF officer's wife. This was seen by some as a job in its own right. Not that I was stereotypical of this breed of woman. For a start I would not alter my behaviour to further my husband's career as so many did. But I had grown up as part of a community and tended to regard each station we inhabited as my community, determined to contribute in whichever way appropriate to its life. So, during my time as a serviceman's wife I ran yoga classes, gave music lessons, was a school governor and a member of the church council. I was called upon to organise floral decorations for functions, to plan and cook lunch parties for upwards of thirty people, and to make after-dinner speeches. From my early thirties people had started to come to me to discuss their problems. I found that deeply satisfying, and it started me along the road of counsellor-training. It was my ambition to train and then practise as a counsellor – but that was for the future. I used to say that listening to and feeding people was what made life worthwhile. It was true that I loved sitting round a table, sharing a meal with family and friends. True too, that I was happiest when in the kitchen preparing a meal. The extent of my love of cooking was to ask for pans for Christmas and birthday presents! Not a very modern female attitude I'm afraid.

So this was my reality. What I was going through must be a nightmare. Mustn't it? Soon I would wake up and all would be well. Wouldn't it? How I wish it were. At first I checked everything that should be familiar. I remember studying Iain's shirts every day as he stood by my bedside in the ITU, to check whether I recognized them. If I was in a dream he would surely wear something weird and wonderful at least one of the days. He didn't. I knew every one. When I was taken by ambulance for various procedures in different hospitals in the town, I would stare out of the window, scanning the passing scenery for familiar streets and shops. There were all too many. Later, when I started going home for the weekend, I followed the route, expecting some strange diversion. How many times had I driven my car along this road? I knew it so well. It hadn't changed. So this was real. I couldn't escape. It was all too real. This dreadful thing really had happened to me.

I still regularly ask myself if this is a bad dream. Can I not go back to the life I know so well – my 'real' life? The answer is always no! I am stuck with this. So too are my family and friends. I shall never be the same again. Nor will they. This is our new reality.

5. More unreality

I was never unconscious. I am told that in all my communication (such as it was) I was perfectly lucid. But looking back the time was full of dreams and hallucinations.

A lot had to do with boats, perhaps because we had a holiday to Orkney with friends booked and were due to go only a couple of weeks after I was taken ill. For several days I entertained the notion that we could cope between us and still go. It was at this point that unreality took over. I imagined that I could be put on the ferry northwards. My in-laws were to be waiting for me on the quay and the plan was that everyone else would disembark and then I would be stretchered off. Everyone did disembark, but no-one came for me. There was nothing I could do but wait. So wait I did. The boat filled up with people and we set off again. Now I began to be troubled. I had been forgotten! Surely I would be offloaded the next time that we arrived! So we turned around and I eagerly anticipated our arrival on the island once again. Imagine my dismay when, yet again I was left on board. This time, someone came and asked me if I would like a 'nice wash' (why are washes always 'nice'?), and proceeded to give me a blanket bath. I never did leave that boat to have my holiday.

A major episode concerning a boat occurred while I was in the High Dependency Unit, and it lasted for quite some time. I was convinced that the hospital was a riverboat. We would travel so far downstream, then stop and come back upstream. We pulled into the side at each end to let people on and off. Big double doors would open at each end of the boat, around which would congregate visitors, patients on trolleys, and members of staff on their way on and off shift. I was quite close to one of these doors and had a good view of the comings and goings. Some people pushed bicycles, some carried heavy baskets; all waited patiently for the doors to open. They could then leave and crowds would surge in. I believed that my visitors came in that way, having parked their cars on the river bank. They would stay until the boat had returned to where they had embarked, and then would take their leave. I remember being confused and bewildered on at least two occasions. On one, Iain had come in, and after a little while realised that he had left something important in the car. He went straight out to get whatever it was. I had visions of him stepping through the doors and falling into the water. Instead he returned minutes later, unscathed, dry, and bringing the mislaid item. How odd! Another time, Iain and the two girls were visiting me. It was time for them to go home. Iain sent the girls to the car ahead of him so that we could have a few moments alone together. I fretted to myself how long it would be until he could get back to the place nearest to where the car was parked, and whether our girls would be all right 'out there' in the dark on their own for that length of time. I never mentioned it and it did not seem to be a problem.

Then there was the medieval hospital. This when I was in the Intensive Care Unit. It was an open room, dark, and full of people; some, like me, were on makeshift beds made up in chairs. Others lay on the floor or on piles of straw. There was a very small door in the opposite wall, through which I would one day escape, I fantasised. Around the corner from my 'bed' slept the resident doctor and her family. She always brought her children with her when she was on duty overnight, and they all slept together in a big brass bed. I was continually pestered by a short, plump woman, trying to sell her services as a nurse. She kept showing me her card, giving me a knowing look, and assuring me that she would look after me well, probably better than anyone else. There was already someone looking after me, and in any case I didn't like her sly, shifty look. She gave me the heebie-jeebies. So I politely explained that I had no need of her services, and she just smiled knowingly and moved on, touting for custom. She never gave up, but regularly came to ask me to take her on. I always gave her the same answer, and she always accepted it. Nevertheless, I was relieved each time I found myself back in my proper place at the other side of the ward, surrounded by familiar and trusted faces.

For a few days I was plagued by dirty cobwebs. These were

all over the ceiling and drifted down constantly. I watched in horrified fascination as the smoke-laden webs came closer and closer to my face. I was powerless to avoid them. I remember thinking that these old NHS buildings really were in a sorry state – and not even clean! Actually, I cannot honestly remember one ever landing on me . . .

At one stage I was involved in the making of a television documentary about young girls taking care of passengers on airliners. Every child had the patter, "Hello, I'm – and I am going to be looking after you during your flight. First I will . . ."

And so it went on. Passengers were invited to change out of their clothes and into some specially designer shell-suits. Their seats were abandoned, and their time was spent in the treatment area at the rear of the plane. There then followed a series of passive exercises, few of which I can remember, and passengers were asked if they needed anything more times than I care to think, after which it was time to get changed ready for the landing. The whole time the girls (for it was all young girls, heavily made up and dressed up to the nines, who participated in this) spoke in a soothing, singsong voice, not unlike those that can be heard over the loudspeaker in the supermarket or department store. I was irritated beyond belief. It all seemed such a waste of time, particularly on the short flights. My frustration grew. But I could only watch and listen. I was very glad when that image faded.

While I was in the Intensive Care Unit, at weekends there would be a tea-party. Each visitor would bring something tasty and all the offerings were added to the food provided by the hospital. Of course we patients did not eat very much, so the visitors had quite a feast. There was much bonhomie and everyone mucked in to do the clearing up. I could watch the proceedings in the kitchen through the big open hatchway. I could see my daughters busying themselves with the platters of food and later the dirty dishes. I, of course, could take no part, but could only lie and watch.

A German family friend had suffered a severe stroke the year before and was very ill. It seemed that he was making no progress. Once again unreality crept in. I dreamt that he came for treatment to the hospital I was in. He brought his wife and a friend with him. His wife, previously of very ample proportions, was incredibly thin – we assumed through the hard work and stress of looking after him at home. The friend, presumably feeling responsible for both of them, was very much in charge. We spent quite a bit of time with them, but he improved more quickly than I did and moved on (he has sadly since died).

My final bizarre account is much less coherent and more difficult to make sense of. Iain and I were travelling around the world. I was flat on my back, paralysed, and needed treatment at each port of call. We had no problems in the poorer countries, but when we reached Australia we had terrible trouble. There, the senior nurse in the casualty department (where I was being seen) was having a flaming row with the doctor who was treating me. I became 'piggy in the middle' and consequently I was not at all well treated. I was very frightened. I also felt very alone. The nurse was intent on getting the better of the doctor and she didn't care who got in her way. I got more and more agitated. The next thing I knew, I was right in the middle of the set of one of those TV hospital dramas. Once again I was afraid – I didn't like the idea of being looked after by actors pretending to be nurses and doctors. There was, however, a medical advisor to the programme, and I depended on her for adequate care. I seemed to be pushed from pillar to post, in the way wherever I was put. I was incredibly relieved when I woke up, for this obviously <u>was</u> a dream!

All this time (and I don't remember how long it was) I was 'talking' lucidly to my family, and as far as I and those who know me were concerned, was quite 'with-it', but looking back, I do wonder whether I was as sensible as I liked to make out. Of course, all these episodes could suggest that I spent the time in and out of sleep. Odd dreams are more acceptable as phenomena than hallucinations, and I like to think that I was quite sane during this time, so my explanation has to be that these were just dreams. They were very unsettling at the time though.

6. The early days

The first three months following the stroke were spent in hospital. I worked my way from the Intensive Care Unit to the High Dependency Unit, and from there to the main ward. I felt dire during my time in Intensive Care. I still had terrible **tinnitus**, and this nearly drove me mad. Actually, it was not so much ringing in my ears as hissing or whooshing – it got louder and softer, reminiscent of breakers crashing onto rocks. But it bore no resemblance to the gentle lapping of waves against the shore, a sound so often associated with relaxation. This relentless noise intruded on every waking moment. I couldn't escape.

Escape of any sort was impossible. I lay immobile, an easy target for all the folk who felt they needed to do things to me. I lost track of the number of needles that were stuck into me. There was daily physiotherapy to my chest, presumably to ensure that I avoided getting pneumonia. Within a few days, two occupational therapists came to make splints for my hands. These were to keep my fingers straight as they were apt to form themselves into tight little fists. I hated those splints. They were hot and uncomfortable and I felt trapped by them.

I felt trapped anyway. There was no way I was going anywhere. I had no control over anything that happened to me. With horror I thought that this was the end of my leisurely breakfasts, reading the newspaper, when the house was empty and quiet. The end, too, of my solitary journeys by car to fetch our daughters home for the holidays, to meet family and friends from the train. Even to go to the supermarket. Gone, too, the happy afternoons and evenings preparing a meal for friends and loved ones and sharing it with them. So much that made up the fabric of my life had disappeared, almost literally overnight. Worst of all, I feared for my marriage. What kind of a wife would I make from now on? I had always considered myself to be a great support to Iain. Now I could only be a burden. And as for physical attraction – I could forget it. That side of things was surely over. I may not be dead but I might just as well be!

I felt very sorry for myself just then, but in the following weeks and months I learned a fair bit about the nature of love, and friendship, and of faith.

The letters and flowers started to flood in. The flowers were brought in for me to see. Then they had to be taken home as they were not allowed in the Intensive Care Unit. I understand that there were so many that they filled our entire stock of vases at home. I wish I had seen the wonderful display they made. The letters were almost unbelievable, not only in the number that arrived, but also in what they said. Everyone who wrote expressed extreme shock at what had happened, and the dreadful unfairness of it. There was also a mountain of cards from neighbours and acquaintances. It struck me that all this correspondence smacked of condolence. *I'm not dead yet* I thought defiantly, as Iain read me all the messages we received. Right from the start, he was intent on keeping me included and informed about everything that concerned us as a family. One of the many letters I received in those early days talked volubly about my 'bereavement'. At first I was affronted. I had narrowly avoided dying and it had been a huge effort! But on reflection, I was grieving the loss (and I continue to do so) of so many things I had, until now, taken for granted. I clung (and still cling) to the hope that they were not gone forever, but were (are) temporarily inaccessible. Hard work and determination would bring them all back. That is what I hoped anyway.

Friends came from far and near to see me, though I only wanted to see the closest of friends and family. Iain and the two girls came every day, and I counted the minutes each morning till they appeared at the door. My mother had stayed on with us and came in with the others most days. Very soon after the stroke Iain's parents arrived, having flown down from the far north. I remember them as two dark figures sitting in the distance; they kept their vigil a little way off. My sister, and Iain's brother and his wife, were regular visitors. My godmother and a handful of my dearest friends were the only other people that I wanted near me. I still had some vanity and was reluctant for people to see me surrounded by machines, with a mass of tubes snaking all over my body and a blank, staring expression on my face. All my loved ones spoke to me as if I was in full possession of my faculties (which of course I was) and kept any feelings of disquiet over my appearance to themselves – something for which I was very grateful.

Iain decided that he should become my advocate. He would point out to all-comers that I was quite 'with it' and should be consulted or informed about everything – the tendency being to address my companion rather than me. I got very irritated at hearing 'she this' and 'she that' when it should have been 'you this' and 'you that'. Iain and I would 'converse' using my eye movements and the alphabet and then he would pass on my wishes or opinions to whomever was concerned.

Looking back, it seems that our 'conversations' were very fluent but in actual fact each exchange was extremely labourious and took an age to execute. We learned to be precise, and although Iain (or whoever was speaking with me) could afford to be expansive, I had to be economical with words, and even with letters. My eyelid got very tired very quickly, and our communication would break down in the absence of a certain degree of accuracy.

In his efforts to keep me included in family affairs, Iain took me on a daily mental tour of the garden. We often used to wander around the garden, frequently with glasses of wine in our hands, examining our collection of plants. We were not great gardeners (although we had plans to be some time in the future!) but we enjoyed our attempts at horticulture. We also enjoyed our little ritual of 'surveying the estate'; it gave Iain a chance to unwind after work and for me it meant a few minutes together in peace and quiet. So Iain tried to recreate that special time in my imagination. He described all that was happening in the garden; all the changes, the triumphs and the disasters. But after a few days of this I could listen no more. I could not bear to hear how good it all looked. I should be there, part of it; not stuck here, unable to move. I might not even see our garden again. Even if I survived, there was no guarantee that I would go home, least of all to that home (RAF Married Quarters) as Iain would shortly be leaving the RAF and we planned to buy our own house. I made it plain that I could not face another mental tour of our garden. That hurt Iain. We both shared the doubts that I would get home.

One evening, Iain tearfully explained his plan for changing our study into a room for my mother. She was currently sharing with Elisabeth, and as she was likely to be staying for some time (at least until I was stable) he thought that it would be a good idea if she had her own room. This would mean, as he pointed out, that the 'office' stuff would have to go in our bedroom, the desk blocking my side of the bed. That would acknowledge, he said tentatively, that I was unlikely to go home – to that house anyway. It did make perfect sense, I had to admit. So, with not a little magnanimity, I gave my blessing to the move and resigned myself to my fate! After several days in Intensive Care I was moved to the High Dependency Unit. I still could only move my left eye up and down and blink; I had a tracheostomy, a nasogastric tube, a urinary catheter and sundry intravenous lines. The latter did have the advantage of sparing me yet more injections. Any drugs I needed could be administered through these lines and the blood so frequently required for testing could be removed via them.

The ratio of nurses to patients in the HDU was almost as high as in ICU so I was rarely alone. The daily round included regular neurological observations (involving amongst other things, shining a torch into my eyes), and two-hourly **nebulisers**. These were little bottles of water fixed on to my tracheostomy. I was still receiving oxygen via my tracheostomy, and it was necessary to humidify it before it entered my lungs. The little bottle was attached to the hose carrying the oxygen, and the water was forced under pressure to mix with the oxygen as I breathed it in. It always made a loud hissing, gurgly sort of noise, and had a distinctive, peppery type of smell. At first I did not mind these little fizzy 'bombs', but later I came to dislike them intensely, because if wrongly positioned or with insufficient pressure going through, they would tip up and deposit their contents down my neck. I ended up with a wet neck all too often!

Much of my time in the HDU was spent watching my fellow patients and making comparisons between our various conditions – wrong, I know. I would note the time that the doctors spent with others compared with their cursory visits to me. Although pleasant, and politeness itself, they always seemed to ask me to do things that were impossible. Things like turning my head, shrugging my shoulders, or stretching out my fingers. I lay resolutely still. My resentment grew around that time. How much more convenient if I had died, I thought. I felt that they did not know what to say to me. They were powerless while my brain tried to right itself.

We had got used to the fact that this was a Serious Business. Our first thoughts had been that this was a tremendous nuisance and would I be well in time for our evening out in London later in the week, or our trip away to celebrate our wedding anniversary the following weekend. Quite soon we had accepted the severity of the situation. The evening out had been cancelled; likewise the weekend away. Now it was time to cancel our holiday. We had arranged to go away with our good friends; everything was booked and paid for. I briefly fretted about letting our friends down, and about retrieving our money, but I was swiftly relieved of that responsibility and, in truth, I had more pressing concerns needing my attention just then.

I looked forward to, nay depended upon, the daily appearance of Iain and the girls. I must give it its due – the RAF was good to us at that time. Iain was given a month's compassionate leave to begin with, and he then worked half-time for a while. Thus he was able to spend lots of time with me. I relied heavily on either Iain or one of the girls being with me. Not least because I felt that with them I would be 'listened-to'. We were perfecting our use of the alphabet for 'conversation'. We were splitting the alphabet in half, on the advice of the rehab consultant (a regular visitor to the severe-stroke patients), with a letter in the first half eliciting a flash of my eyes heavenward, and one in the second half a look downwards. We as a family were soon quite proficient at this method of communication. Iain started keeping a notebook in which my 'utterances' were noted. This performed two functions: namely, it helped the 'listener' keep track of sentences as they emerged, and it allowed me to continue using the vocabulary to which I was accustomed. Long and complicated words needed to be written down as they materialised so that the beginning was not forgotten by the time I got to the end. I took a perverse delight in using the most complicated words I could muster, and watching the expressions on the scribes' faces as they tried to work out what was coming. As the days wore on Iain began to hand the notebook to visiting friends. This was met with a countenance of complete trepidation. It was evidently an awesome responsibility! Whoever held the notebook 'ran' the conversation; all eyes (including mine) turned to that person. Some people found it quite daunting; some got lost very quickly – I was quite amused by the number of people who got in a muddle when reciting the alphabet. At least we could laugh together, if not talk together. Others took to it readily, and although the procedure was incredibly slow, I did feel that I was having some sort of a conversation with them. I indicated that I had something to say, whether it be a casual remark or a request, by a quick up and down flash of my eyes. This was of course all dependent upon other people attending closely to me. I was always at the mercy of other people's goodwill and interest. The passive nature of my position was all too evident. This just compounded it.

One major concern was that there was no way I could call a nurse. We felt very optimistic when we heard that the speech therapist specialising in communication aids was coming to see me. She arrived, carrying her wares in a large plastic box, and proceeded to unpack all sorts of communication aids. One by one they were deemed unsuitable, as my eyes were the only part of me that I could use (and they only moved up and down), while the aids needed lateral eye movements as well. She brought things such as big alphabet charts (where you gaze at the letter you require), and other charts, similar to the one I was able to use in casualty, which needed the use of a finger to point, and an electronic gadget which synthesized a voice speaking the word typed in. We then moved on to the problem of calling the nurse.

"If only she could move her head," the lady sighed to Iain (a good example of people with the infuriating habit of talking about me rather than to me! I would have loved to make some stinging remark but of course I remained silent). If I could have moved my head I could have had a switch on my pillow which, with momentary pressure from my head, would ring a bell to summon a nurse. If only . . . lots of things! Of course if I could do more it would make life easier. We needed help to cope with things as they were! We were not impressed! The lady left with her box of goodies. Nothing had changed. Fortunately, the technician had a different attitude. He came to see me a few days later with a pair of spectacles in his hand. They were fitted with a switch, operated by the blinking of my eye. I was captivated by the ability to make something work, after so long of lying doing nothing. The spectacles, however, were big and unwieldy and I was unable, of course, to adjust them once they were on. Privately, as those around me discussed ways of using them effectively, I decided that by the time the spectacles were sorted out, I would not need them. Rash and optimistic!

It was around this time that my sister came up with the idea of the 'body service'. All the little personal 'maintenance' tasks that I would have carried out privately (such as shaving my armpits and legs) were covered by this expression, and my sister offered to take care of them. I was extremely grateful for this offer, if rather embarrassed. She was helped by one of my daughters, and set about the 'service' with great aplomb. While I have been incapable of doing these things for myself, it has been a relief that either my sister or one of my daughters was keeping an eye on such matters for me.

My day consisted at this time of 'total patient care'. I was washed from head to toe in bed, and was turned regularly from side to back, to prevent problems from excessive, prolonged pressure. The **tracheostomy tube** in my neck was connected by a big hose to the oxygen supply and my throat had to be suctioned out through it frequently because of the ferocious coughing fits I experienced. My poor throat was irritated not only by the mucus and other 'junk' that collected there, but also by the tube itself (in fact, years after the tube was removed, my throat is still intolerant of the slightest irritation). Back in the Intensive Care Unit the dietician had calculated the number of calories per day I needed and I received these in the form of two types of disgusting-smelling liquid. These were pumped into my stomach via a nasogastric tube, as eating and drinking were out of the question. This was my meat and two veg, and it was washed down with the required amount of water. In my years of nursing, I had inserted many such tubes – up inside one nostril and bending round to come down the back of the throat and on into the stomach. I had always acknowledged that it was unpleasant but really, I had had no idea! The tube was anchored to the nose with sticking plaster, and that in itself was uncomfortable – in addition to giving one the look of an elephant, the 'trunk' dangling down in front of one's face! But having one passed, as I did a few times owing to it being inadvertently pulled out, was absolutely vile. Nowadays, they use an 'introducer' – a long straight piece of metal which fitted inside the tube to ensure that it is kept straight on its way down to the stomach. It is fairly rigid, so getting it round the corner at the top of the nose, in order to go down the oesophagus (via the nasopharynx of course) was not easy and consequently not pleasant. It tended to scratch the throat on the way down and that – in addition to the almost inevitable coughing and retching that accompanied the procedure – ensured that it was a thoroughly ghastly experience. When it was in place the ordeal was not over, for there was the constant feeling of discomfort and irritation at the back of the throat, often provoking the reflex to expel it.

"It would be much better if you had a gastrostomy," said the wise doctors on their flying visits. Well, true enough, it *would* be nice to get rid of the tube up my nose. Instead, there would be a tube going directly through the skin into my stomach via which the liquid food could be pumped. It was a fairly common procedure for the long-term feeding of people who for one reason or another were unable to eat.

There was a problem however. Since the endotracheal tube had been removed and replaced by the tracheostomy, my jaw had become progressively tighter, and now my mouth was firmly shut. The teeth were clenched, and nothing short of brute force was likely to open it. The customary procedure for putting in these gastrostomy tubes was to pass a fibre-optic 'telescope' through the mouth, down into the stomach where the tube could be introduced through the skin and anchored 'under supervision'. This would not work with me. For a start, the 'telescope' would not have got into my mouth, let alone any further, so it was decided that a new and different procedure should be carried out. I was put on the waiting list for an insertion of gastrostomy tube under radiological control.

Of course I had an array of intravenous lines in addition to all this. The 'drips' had come down and a couple of the lines were soon removed. The rest remained to be used for the administration of drugs. This was an efficient route for giving drugs unless the **cannula** got blocked. I dreaded the signs – the nurse trying repeatedly to push the syringe full of liquid through, and muttering frustratedly under her breath. I hated the idea of having a line replaced; I had had enough needles stuck in me already. Imagine my relief when she 'fiddled' and managed to unblock the tube and the threat receded!

It was troubling me that the birthdays of some of our friends and relations were looming closer. It was always my job (by default) to remember the various anniversaries throughout the year. If I didn't remember no-one else would. Attracting attention was the next challenge. We had worked out that a repeated flashing of my eyes up and down meant 'I want to say something' or 'I need something'. Then I had to spell out the request for a birthday card, and the message to go in it. It was duly done as I instructed, and this procedure was repeated for the next few months. It was quite a revelation to those around me that my memory was intact; another assurance that 'I was still in there'.

I was still having weird dreams, most of which involved people I knew and which often included some form or other of recovery for me. What an optimist! Despite this, I continued to be sane yet silent, alert though inactive.

As during my stay in the Intensive Care and High Dependency Units I was not allowed any flowers but yet they kept pouring in: they were whisked off home. They made, I am told, a fantastic display the like of which the house has not seen before or since. Also during this time the number of visitors allowed around my bedside at any given time was limited. This meant that our daughters spent a great deal of time in the relatives' sitting room outside the ward. Since some quiet occupation was needed, Elisabeth was forced to read and revise her schoolwork. This paid dividends; when her GCSEs came around later in the year, despite the huge upheaval in the rest of her life she excelled herself. Those hours spent in silent solitude reaped their reward. For that we must be thankful.

Soon the visiting medical staff began muttering about moving me to the main ward.

"It will be so much nicer for you," they kept saying. I had my doubts. Up until now I almost had a nurse to myself. I depended on each one to be a mind-reader, or at least an excellent observer; to sense or to see my needs. On the main ward I would have to share the staff with twenty or so others – and I could not expect my own private mind-reader. Of course this was progress but I was scared.

7. Moving on

The day dawned when I was to be moved to the main ward. In the event though, the day was nearly over by the time the transfer was finally made. Iain offered to stay overnight by my side. That was such a relief. I was so frightened – more so than I had been during the previous weeks. I always felt reassured, though, whenever Iain or the girls were with me. So I was settled into my new surroundings and Iain settled down in a comfortable chair by my side. Thus began the next phase of my so-called recovery; the acute, crisis time was over and the hard slog was about to begin.

Throughout this whole business I have felt as if I were two people: one extremely objective, interested, and at times critical, and the other very worried, passive and despondent. It seemed to be a conversation opener that I had been a nurse, and I was glad of that. It seemed to give me some identity. I was 'one of us', worthy of some recognition. Of course I understood what had happened inside my brain and I knew (but preferred not to consider) the long-term implications. I also had some experience of caring for people with similar problems and had my own ideas of what constituted good nursing care. I was fascinated, if a little dismayed, to see the changes that had occurred over the years since I had left nursing. Twenty years ago, the mainstay of the workforce (for better or worse!) was the student nurse. The qualified staff were less numerous, more knowledgeable (or so it seemed) and vastly more experienced than their modern counterparts. Now there were trained staff everywhere, and students were few and far between. There was nothing to distinguish the recently-qualified from the experienced staff nurses. Nothing, that is, except their demeanour. The 'newer' staff nurses were noticeably less confident and less competent than their more mature colleagues – worryingly so in some cases. There were technical issues: the nurse who put my drugs in the wrong tube of my gastrostomy and burst the retaining balloon, and the one who tried to suck out my tracheostomy with the suction catheter wrongly connected. But there were also communication and organisational problems; the older nurses were generally more patient, more concerned with my comfort and attentive to detail. I looked out for certain members of staff being on duty, for then I knew that all would be well. The critical part of me observed and assessed the comings and goings on the ward. Being judgmental has always been one of my biggest faults. The other part of me, however, sought reassurance, hoping that someone 'good' – both competent and kind – was around or waiting anxiously for Iain or the girls to come in. I felt better when they were with me. They tended to take 'shifts' throughout the day, one or other of them coming in at about ten in the morning. If I was uncomfortable or bothered about something, I would reassure myself with the thought that they would soon be in and thus stay relatively calm.

First thing in the morning was blanket-bath time. I felt like a beached whale, lying there unclothed, tubes protruding from various orifices, and being washed all over. Quite often, when the nurses rolled me over to wash my back, I would catch sight of my reflection in the bedside mirror. I was appalled at what I saw. That bloated face, with unkempt hair plastered to it, and tiny, staring eyes – that surely was not me? Was it? There was a hole in the neck (quite often with a green plastic hose appearing to come from it) and a long thin tube dangling from the nose. With a mixture of horror and despair I had to admit to myself that it really was me. I resolved to avoid seeing myself in the mirror any more and to prevent any wider circle of friends and acquaintances coming to see me.

The ward staff could be divided into two groups: those I trusted and those I did not. I grew to depend on the former so much; they were attentive and observant. They treated me as an intelligent human being, whatever the creature in the bed resembled. Best of all, they seemed to be able to read my mind; I could rely on them to know my needs and to meet them. One of these was the ward's Health Care Assistant (HCA). A woman of about my age, I developed an almost childlike dependency on her. It was she who, more often than not, would wash me in the morning, notice when I was uncomfortable and straighten me up, and rescue me when I coughed myself dangerously near the edge of the bed.

Coughing was a tremendous problem for many months following the stroke and, to a lesser extent, still is. Of course there are those who would not regard it as such. A strong cough reflex helps to protect the airway – that being a most important consideration, and an obsession of anaesthetists, physiotherapists, speech therapists and nurses. To me, the cough was a real trial; causing discomfort, worry and, worst of all for me, embarrassment. It was ironic that, paralysed as I was, involuntary actions such as coughing, yawning or sneezing could provoke quite big movements. Coughing would often send me bouncing across the bed and, not infrequently, leave me perilously close to, or just over, the edge. There I would hang, strangely enough not panicking, waiting patiently to be rescued. Someone would eventually notice my predicament and straighten me up.

When one has a tracheostomy, troublesome secretions are suctioned out of the area of the throat via the tracheostomy tube. When I was nursing, the whole business of looking after a tracheostomy tube filled me with trepidation. Even passing the long, thin suction tube down inside the tracheostomy tube into the throat was quite a skilled task, not to be undertaken lightly. Yet, having been shown how to do it once, our daughters were able to suck me out after each coughing fit, and even seemed confident at it. This was one among many skills that the family learned and undertook frequently and without complaint during the ensuing months.

It was Easter soon after I arrived on the ward. I had no Easter eggs for anyone! What was I to do? In the past, I had always tried to make things a bit special at Easter-time but that would not be happening this year. But the least I could do would be to get eggs for everyone. So, with my eyes, I asked Elisabeth to do my shopping for me. I gave her a list of whom to buy for – including herself – and she duly brought in the necessary goodies. Fortunately I had some cash in my purse to give her for the shopping – the last vestige of my independence. Easter Sunday was very strange. All the family came in, of course, and we exchanged Easter eggs and gifts, but there the similarity with our usual Easters ended. There was no big family roast lunch (cooked by me of course), no sticky chocolate cake for tea. I was not part of the decorating team at church and for the first time in many years I missed the Easter services. The hospital chaplain came and said some prayers at my bedside. He was a regular visitor; however, I found his visits rather tiresome. He seemed to favour long silences and these make me feel most uncomfortable. I was familiar with the counselling technique of maintaining prolonged silences to encourage a client to be the one to break them with his thoughts. But I was no client, and I was incapable of breaking any silence. I suspected, rather uncharitably, that he simply did not know what to say to me. Either way, I did not like it one bit and was always relieved when the visits were over. Mercifully there were plenty of calls on his time that day, so we heard a small part of the Easter service and there was no time for long silences.

I was not eating at this stage, so chocolate eggs were out of the question for me. Instead Iain came up with the idea of giving me, of all things, two small soft toy bears. This was in fact a brainwave. The splints which had been made for my hands, to keep my fingers extended, were very uncomfortable. Consequently I would only tolerate wearing them for extremely short periods of time, and for the majority of the time I had tight little fists. My fingernails bore into my palms and gouged angry-looking marks. The bears were the ideal solution. My fingers were prised out straight and were wrapped around the bears, the thumb and forefingers around each neck. As my hands became tenser, the grip around their necks became tighter; thus I was encouraged, by family and staff alike, to 'strangle the bears'. The poor creatures soon became quite deformed; their necks becoming elongated, and their heads peering at people from the strangest of angles. These bears became essential items of equipment. Named Lucas and Rufus by Elinor (for obvious reasons), they became my close companions for many months to come.

Easter was another occasion when I was inundated with flowers. This time I was allowed to keep them. Beautiful bouquets and baskets of spring flowers kept arriving for me, some from the most surprising people, and I derived great pleasure from them. Soon more tables had to be brought in on which to display them, and I very quickly earned a reputation for having a florist's shop around my bed. I never tired of receiving them, and continued to get a buzz out of seeing someone with an armful of flowers looking for me.

Something else that I received in quantity around that time was the evidence of people's different faiths. I received many notes and messages from people who said that they were praying for me. Not only that, but various groups of people, many of whom I had never met, were remembering me in their prayers or thinking about me in their own particular way. One of my friends reported that I was the focus of attention at her mother's coffee-mornings. I found it all rather humbling. Another friend wrote to say that she felt quite helpless, but what she could do would be to hold a special Mass in my name. So she did! At that point two things hit home hard. One was the severity of the situation; there was little anyone could do except Watch and Pray, Live and Hope, depending on their particular beliefs. The other was that so many people cared about what was happening to me. Letter after letter, message after message; expressions of shock, horror and support (some from people with whom we had had no contact for a while) arrived continually. I was astounded, and I derived tremendous comfort from the sheer scale of the concern. I resolved again to fight. I was not alone!

Soon after Easter I was due to have my gastrostomy. Because my mouth was clamped tight shut, the usual procedure for guiding the tube correctly into the stomach (via an endoscope passed through the mouth and down the oesophagus) was impossible. So a new procedure was to be tried. The tube was to be inserted straight into the stomach, through the abdominal wall, with the guidance of a constant x-ray picture. As this procedure could not be carried out at my hospital, I had to go by ambulance to a different hospital on the other side of the city. Iain came with me. He was at my side each time I had to undergo any sort of unpleasant procedure. For this I was extremely grateful. In addition to the comfort I felt from having my husband with me, I gained considerable confidence from knowing that he understood what was going on, was keeping a watchful eye on what was happening to me, and was not afraid to speak up if the need arose (whether Iain felt that confident I don't know, but the thought that he did gave me a measure of strength!). He always did the communicating for me, and I trusted him implicitly to state my case. The inability to speak up for myself would have been more horrifying had he not been with me.

The ambulance men came to collect me. They immediately irritated me by calling me by my Christian name instead of 'Mrs Cromarty'. They were not the only ones to do this. Throughout the eighteen months that I spent in various institutions, and afterwards, I was irritated by the custom of the majority of healthcare workers at all levels of calling people (patients and staff alike) by their first names. They rarely asked how I preferred to be addressed, and even if I did express a preference for being addressed more formally, there was often the implication that they thought I was stand-offish, or even a snob. Only very occasionally did I meet someone with similar old-fashioned principles, who was sufficiently self-confident not to confuse respect with subservience. Of course I met a lot of people during those many months with whom it became natural to be on first name terms. I became very close to some of them and we became firm friends. But I particularly objected to first name familiarity from complete strangers, and especially from the teenagers frequently sent by the agencies to make up the complement of ward staff.

Well, I was collected from the ward by the ambulance crew, and we set off along the maze of corridors to the ambulance. How strange I felt as we sped along, strapped as I was to that hard trolley, staring up at the ceiling, watching the lights whizz past, until we reached the vehicle; there I was slid into place, fastened down, and so began the journey across the city to the hospital where I would have the tube fitted.

I didn't recognise the streets we travelled along; this was a part of town I didn't know. Cars, pedestrians, shops and houses all flashed by. I wasn't concentrating on any of it, and there was a general air of unreality about it all. Suddenly I caught sight of a Park and Ride bus. The sort of bus I had used many times; I tended to leave my car outside the city when I came to shop. Those buses were, to me, synonymous with special shopping days out, forays to the market, or Christmas trips.

A horrible sick feeling came over me as I realised that I was unlikely to travel on those buses again. No more of the solitary shopping trips to buy surprises for the family. No more running up the double-decker bus stairs to sit at the very front with my daughters like three giggly children. In short, no more of the life I was used to!

I burst into tears. Silent tears, because my vocal cords didn't work, but my heart broke nonetheless.

Yet another maze of corridors, and I was in the endoscopy suite. Nurses bustled about, technicians adjusted and moved equipment, and the whole place seemed to hum with weird machinery. I was glad to have Iain by my side. I felt that he would protect me, and more importantly, speak for me since I could not speak up for myself.

The doctor who was to carry out the procedure explained all about it and went on to say that he preferred patients to stay awake during it. My heart skipped a beat! I was not prepared for this! Then I heard Iain saying that I tended to make involuntary movements and it couldn't be guaranteed that I would lie still. In that case, it was decided, I would be heavily sedated while the hole was bored through into my stomach. What a relief! For once I was thankful for the twitches and spasms which, with the coughing, made me leap uncontrollably around the bed. The thought of being awake while my abdomen was punctured made my blood run cold! But fortunately I would not have to face that. Something I did have to face though was the passing of another nasogastric tube. I thought I had avoided that. During the previous night, my existing tube had come out by itself. It had not immediately been replaced. *Oh good*, I had thought, *the gastrostomy will go in tomorrow. I won't need another of those.*

I was wrong. I lay still while another tube was pushed up my nose, scraped the back of my throat, and ended up in my stomach. It was apparently required so that air could be blown into my stomach. An inflated organ, they told me, makes an easier target to aim for. So, a tedious period of what seemed like 'fiddling about' followed, as my stomach was blown up and the optimum position found. All this was done with the help of x-ray guidance. It would have been fascinating watching my innards working, had I not felt a combination of severe discomfort at what was being done to me, and fear of what would happen next.

I can't be sure what did happen next, because at that point I was sedated. I knew nothing until I came to. Iain and I were being told what to expect, and what to do now that the gastrostomy tube was in position and ready to be used. It was tethered by two long wires – sutures, the doctor called them although they didn't look like sutures to me when I eventually saw them. Sutures to me meant threads, these were iron-mongery. They would be cut in ten days, the theory being that they would fall into my intestine, and be passed out in the usual way! There was a large dressing over the site, and I felt very sore. We had an inordinately long wait for an ambulance to take me back. I was thoroughly sore and fed-up. Eventually, however, the ambulance arrived and we made the journey back. I was extremely relieved when I was back in my bed, another unpleasant experience behind me.

8. Improvements?

I hated night-time. During the day, there were comings and goings: visitors, jobs to be done and, crucially, one or more of my family with me. Although I couldn't move or communicate with most people, the fact that I could 'converse' with Iain and my two daughters meant that when they were with me I didn't feel completely helpless. But they would do my exercises, settle me down for the night and then go home for some well-earned food and rest. Then I felt really alone. The curtains were drawn, the lights lowered, the day staff came to say goodnight, and the long, lonely night began. I had my back to the nurses' station. I could hear the night staff assembling for duty. They chatted, laughed and joked. The phone rang, and was answered with cries of "it's for you." More laughter. I lay and listened, willing someone, anyone, to come and see me.

I was lying on an air mattress, which regularly altered the pressure it exerted on each part of my body, in an effort to prevent pressure sores developing. In addition, I was turned every two hours. From my back I was moved to each side in turn. On my back I was reasonably comfortable – for this was the position in which I usually slept. But within a couple of minutes of being put on my side, I felt uncomfortable. Bits of me ached, itched, or felt squashed. I was totally paralysed, so I could not alter my position, but my sensation was almost completely intact. Two hours felt interminable. Of course I had no way of calling a nurse. I could not even call out as one passed. Instead I cultivated a look of anguish in the hope that someone would notice me in passing, take pity on me and move me before my time was up.

There were other reasons for attending to me at night, for which I was extremely thankful. Firstly there was my feed. I had a continuous regime of liquid food and water administered at first via my nasogastric tube, and subsequently through the gastrostomy. Every few hours the bottle would need changing. A nurse would be summoned by the bleeping of the electric pump used to encourage the fluid along the tube. Another reason for coming to my bedside was to administer the eye drops which were applied regularly throughout the night. My right eye wouldn't close properly, so in order to give it some protection, synthetic tears were put into my eye every few hours. Most nurses would gently close my eye for me when I wanted to sleep. It would stay closed for a little while, then gradually creep open again. So the process would have to be repeated again and again. Lastly, as I was taking nothing orally, my mouth had to be cleaned and freshened regularly day and night.

At night some of the nurses were more assiduous about this than others. Of course how often I was visited for these smaller tasks depended a lot on the other pressures on the staff, but however frequent the visits, it was not enough for me. I felt very vulnerable and lonely at night. Iain sensed my unease and offered to stay with me one night a week. He chose Fridays, because our daughters could then relieve him on Saturday morning and he could go home to freshen up, eat, and catch up on sleep if necessary. I was over the moon. From now on at least I could depend on one comfortable night in seven. I would have Iain at my bedside all night. He who knew that I was still an intelligent human being, he who understood me, he who had time for me. I looked forward to Fridays. The girls were with me all day, and in the evening Iain would take over, stay the night, and on into the morning until he was relieved by Elinor and Elisabeth. Later, the Easter holiday over, we decided that Elisabeth ought to go back to boarding school. The crisis seemed to be over. It was now just a case of taking one day at a time, working at everything to get as much back as possible. Besides, Elisabeth had important exams ahead; her GCSEs were only weeks away. She really must get back into the thick of things. I was concerned that the strain of the past weeks, plus the upheaval in our normally well-ordered family life, would have affected her badly and her results might reflect this. As it turned out I needn't have worried, but at that stage the effect all this might have on our daughters was one of my greatest concerns. So Iain took Elisabeth back to school, and a small amount of normality was reintroduced into our family's daily life. My mother went home, with the promise of a daily phone call so that she could keep abreast of everything that was going on. Elinor went back to work as a health care assistant at our local general hospital. She reduced her hours so that she could carry on spending time with me. Iain was to work half days, with the blessing of his RAF boss, so that he too could spend as much time as possible at the hospital. In time, Elinor too offered to stay overnight at my bedside, so then on two nights a week I could count on a worry-free sleep. I did look forward to those two nights a week!

My attention span was very short around this time, and I became very self-interested and self-centred. I had previously held a keen interest in current affairs, and frequently worried about others' well-being, especially the safety of my family. But now I just didn't have the energy to concentrate on any of these things. There were atrocities being perpetrated in the Balkans, and the murder of people (famous and otherwise) in this country, but it all went right over my head. I really couldn't be bothered with such things, if indeed I believed that they were real. As for family members' safety, I just didn't have the wherewithal to worry. Each night, as they left, I just trusted that they would appear the next day. It was not until many months later that I started seeking telephone reassurance that they had arrived home safely. As for my attention, it became most noticeable on Friday evenings that I very quickly lost concentration and interest in things. Friday was the night that Iain spent with me, and we would settle down mid-evening to watch television. This had been another of our rituals at home; for us, certain TV programmes on a Friday night had heralded the weekend. It was therefore quite important that we carry on this tradition in hospital. We clutched at straws of 'normality' wherever we could find them. So we duly put on the TV, and took great comfort and pleasure in the familiar tunes and programmes which for so long had signalled our time together. But, a few minutes later I had had enough. The words spoken became an unintelligible buzz, and I couldn't focus on the picture. This should have been the high spot of the week, but it took too much effort. All I had energy and attention for was simply existing. I was trying to defy this thing that had rendered me helpless, but so far I was having little success.

'This thing' held an awful fascination for us both. Iain bought books on the subject and trawled the internet for medical papers and accounts of research – for this was no 'ordinary' stroke! Time has taught me that there is no such thing as an 'ordinary' stroke. Just as every individual is unique, so each 'insult' to the brain – complex structure that it is – is unique and can affect its victim in a myriad of different ways. Iain would read research papers to me, quoting statistics, giving me hope and despair alternately as I compared myself with the subjects of these accounts. I soon realised the folly of this, and determined not to follow those documented patterns. *I'll prove them all wrong*, I thought defiantly (this has proved much more difficult than I imagined!). One paper listed the possible effects of stroke – in addition to the obvious ones such as paralysis. One was 'inappropriate laughter'. Victims would laugh, often uncontrollably, at the most inappropriate times, and in totally unsuitable situations.

Oh no, I thought, *that's not me*. I react to things that are vaguely amusing with, at most, a wry smile. My sense of humour is much too dry to allow that sort of behaviour'!

How wrong I was! It wasn't long before I started giggling at the most unfunny people and situations. I felt so ashamed. I knew what was happening, knew it was totally inappropriate, but could do nothing about it. I didn't speak, so explanations were obviously out of the question. On the one hand, this was a reaction from someone who had previously been totally unresponsive, so it was welcomed and encouraged by some members of staff. But on the other it quickly became an irritation to some, because I apparently did not know when to stop. I knew when to stop all right – and when not to start! I just had no control over it. I was at the mercy of my involuntary behaviour, and had to suffer in silence as I was regarded as at best a little odd and at worst completely deranged. Even after eighteen months, I still laughed when I was irritated or worried, and grinned when appalled or sad. There seemed little that I could do about it. Now, as then, it makes me furious with myself.

Laughter was not the only involuntary behaviour I had. Paralysed though I might be, there was also the frequent cough which could move me phenomenal distances. My limbs would leap high off the bed. Unfortunately, I couldn't reproduce these movements at will and they were totally uncontrollable. I often found myself alarmingly close to the edge of the bed, completely unable to right myself! I just had to wait until someone passed and noticed my predicament. I also had a very wide yawn. Most of the time my jaws were clamped tight shut. But when I yawned my mouth opened cavernously wide – again without warning or control – and closed just as suddenly, returning to its vicelike condition. Often I would catch my tongue or my cheek between my teeth as they guillotined down. I could not stop the remorseless bite, and the hapless piece of mouth would be trapped and squashed. It was agony! I soon had an extremely sore mouth, and came to dread that telltale feeling of a yawn brewing.

Looking back at this time, it seems that Iain and I had long conversations, but in fact we were still using our 'eye-flash' method of communication. We had become quite slick at this. Dividing the alphabet in two, and writing my 'utterances' down, to keep track of things helped to make the whole procedure relatively speedy. To an outsider it was awe-inspiring, and the uninitiated blanched when they were handed 'the book' (and so were in control of the conversation) and took the responsibility very seriously.

It was about this time that Elinor announced that she did not want to go to university, but intended staying at home to look after me. I was horrified! The previous year we had all been dreadfully disappointed when rejection after rejection from medical schools had arrived. But in the weeks preceding my stroke she had received unconditional offers from no less than three places. As far as I was concerned, Elinor's immediate future was secure. The only unknown factor was which place she would choose. Now it seemed that she was going to throw it away. I was very touched of course, but it could not be allowed. How was I going to deliver a stern motherly lecture with 'eye-flashes'? For I felt that the protest had to come from me and be as strong as possible. I felt panic-stricken at the thought of her throwing it all in and becoming my nursemaid. What was to happen to me I had no idea. I breathed through a tube, was fed via a tube, and passed urine through a tube.

From where I lay, going home seemed almost impossible, but of one thing I was sure: our daughters would not be prevented, by anything that happened to me, from pursuing the futures they had planned. So I began my protest.

A frantic flashing up and down of my eyelids indicated that I had something to 'say'. The distress must have been evident as I spelled out my feelings about Elinor abandoning her plans for medical school. I was very fortunate that my family and friends took notice of the signs that I wanted to 'speak', and of what I had to 'say' (even if they didn't like what came across). It would have been so easy to ignore. This was a very passive form of communication, and I always felt at the mercy of the 'listener'. Elinor took note of my feelings, her face set in a stubborn mask, but over time we managed to persuade her to try university just for a year. She chose the one the furthest south of the three, in the hope that it would be the closest to home – wherever that was to be.

I was visited daily by two physiotherapists. The junior of the two would exercise and stretch my limbs and joints. There is a very real danger that a stroke victim's joints will seize up and deformities result through lack of use and the repeated spasms in the affected limbs. These exercises and muscle stretches were designed to combat this, and were carried out twice a day. I enjoyed these passive movements. I exercised and stretched a lot in my yoga classes and liked the feeling of ease-of-movement that I had. There was no spontaneous movement now, so it was very pleasant to feel the bending and stretching of my joints and muscles. So I was content to relax and let this young lady carry on with her work. From time to time she worried that she might be causing me pain. She wasn't. Contrary to what some people suggested, I had not lost the feeling in my body, only the voluntary movement. My years of yoga had left my joints sufficiently supple to tolerate, and even enjoy, the movements which they were put through. I have since been told that I have not experienced the contractures and deformities that experts expect from a stroke of this severity because of my general high level of suppleness. Yet another reason to be grateful to yoga. The senior physiotherapist came along a little later, bringing the 'tilt table' with her. Every day I was slid onto this, strapped to it, and taken up to the vertical. Once there, I had to exercise the parts of my body that were 'waking up'. I regularly had a coughing fit while up there, which provoked a mixed reaction of horror and amusement. I was securely strapped in position, so I didn't worry too much, although on a couple of occasions I did begin to feel very faint. The physiotherapists must have noticed, for I was then whisked down and put back to bed pretty smartly.

Those two ladies were the greatest source of professional encouragement while I was in hospital, and were the best of all the physiotherapists I encountered during my so-called recovery. They always treated me with a mixture of friendliness and respect; of considerable importance since my self-respect lay in tatters. As each new little movement returned, I would show them with great pride. They shared my excitement, however small the muscle was that was twitching, and however useful or useless the movement was likely to be. The stars of the show were my head and neck, which slowly gained in strength and flexibility. It was not too long before I could manage a lopsided smile, and nod and shake my head.

I could also control the movements of my head sufficiently to allow me to use a pillow-switch. This meant I could call the nurse. What a difference that made! I no longer felt so isolated. I worried less about whether there was a nurse nearby; I could call one if I needed her. The day dawned when they announced that there was a hospital wheelchair for me. This was to be a temporary arrangement so that I could sit out and be pushed around the hospital. In due course, a wheelchair was brought in, together with a hoist with which to put me into it. Lifting me out of bed and putting me in the wheelchair was a major undertaking. The first time it involved the two physiotherapists and two or three nurses. I was hoisted up in the air with great care and attention. The sling in which I was attached to the hoist was put around me with great care, and a nurse was detailed to support my head. The hoist was raised, and I swung across from the bed, and into the chair. I was lowered very gingerly into it, and placed very carefully with my back and limbs arranged 'in a good position'. The chair was tipped back, so that gravity would help to keep me in the chair – sitting up straight was completely out of the question. I was like a rag doll; totally floppy, and unable to support my own weight. The various tubes emanating from my body had to be moved carefully with me and put in place, so that they still worked. The physiotherapists then set about adjusting various parts of the chair to 'ensure a good fit'.

How I hated that chair! I hated all that it stood for. It seemed to scream out, 'Look at me, I am disabled'! I felt that it was a badge, announcing to the world that my body didn't work, and perhaps my mind didn't either. While I lay (or was propped up) in bed, I could kid myself that I was temporarily ill, that I could at any time just throw back the covers and, perhaps with a little help, climb out of bed. The ignominy of being hoisted into a wheelchair put paid to that. There was no escape! I had become disabled! I vowed silently that I would soon discard this, and although I did not expect to regain my previous level of activity, I intended to surprise everyone by getting up and about, doing things, however small, around the place.

I developed quite a chip on my shoulder. People had better not assume that because my body was paralysed, my mind was too. I looked out constantly for patronising behaviour and, more often than not, found it. The inappropriate and uncontrollable laughter from which I suffered didn't help. I was so often humoured and treated as a harmless but unintelligent child. I felt both mortified and livid. How dare people treat me like that – but didn't my involuntary behaviours just encourage it?

I was thus forced to confront and examine my own prejudices. 'The disabled' were a distinct group, separate from the rest of the population. They needed various aids, and in some cases people, to do what they wanted – to lead 'a full life'! Hadn't I made a study of provisions for 'the disabled'? I understood their needs, and their wishes to be independent. But I was happy to get on with my life; paying no attention to the number of steps I had to climb in shops, restaurants and even private houses. It took a matter of moments to leap out of bed in the morning, shower, put on my makeup, do my hair, and put on my clothes, however complicated. I could drive to the shops, push open the doors, reach the shelves, read the labels, chat to the shop assistant, and sign my name on the credit card slip. I never gave a thought to those for whom these everyday tasks caused difficulty. Any consideration I did give to 'those poor unfortunate people' was either academic or thankfulness that my life was untouched by such 'inconvenience'. This was a group of people separate and distant from me. Some would engender embarrassment in others, either by their appearance or by some aspect of their behaviour; children would stare and ask awkward questions; and they were given special consideration, and even special facilities in some places and at some functions. In short, 'they' were different.

And here was I, being hoisted into a wheelchair. I couldn't move or talk. The professionals around me talked of 'this aid' or 'that aid' and there was talk of my being Registered Disabled. Disabled? I screamed inside: *I am not disabled. I am ME! That hasn't changed! My limbs might not work; my voice doesn't. My eyes and my lungs don't work properly; and I don't eat or drink. But hey, I'm still me. That hasn't changed. My memory is just as sharp as ever; my wit still as cruel (perhaps it was just as well sometimes that I was unable to give vent to it!), and I am still intolerant of fools (and particularly those who treat me like one!). In short, I am just the same, an individual with unique qualities; my 'only' problem is that my body won't work.*

As I lay festering with frustration and anger about this, I realised with shame that I was not alone in feeling that way. 'The Disabled', a term convenient for lumping people with problems together, were individuals just like me. Each had strengths and weaknesses, likes and dislikes, principles and prejudices of his or her own. Why regard 'them' as so different from 'us'? Throughout the time since my stroke I have resisted fiercely the notion of being known as 'disabled', while at the same time feeling ashamed of myself for harbouring such a patronising and ignorant attitude.

The plan was that I should sit out in the wheelchair for increasingly long periods. Then I could be wheeled to places; the garden, for instance, or around and about the hospital. There were (at least) two problems with this, as far as I was concerned. I dribbled. A continuous stream of saliva trickled from my mouth. Of course with hindsight it is straightforward to explain. I was sitting up (after a fashion) and I couldn't send the saliva backwards to my throat (my tongue didn't work), nor swallow it automatically (that didn't work properly either), so out it came. I felt mortified. I hate to think what it looked like. I thought that if I ignored it, it might go away. Of course it didn't. I dribbled like a teething baby. Visiting friends came armed with boxes of tissues. Someone was constantly wiping my face. I wanted to hide it. The second problem was caused by the persistent, violent, cough. Every time I coughed, the upper part of my body would lurch forward and fill everyone with alarm – not least me! It seemed as though I would launch myself head first out of the chair. This called for some serious thought; there was much scratching of heads. The problem was not so great when there was a table in front of the chair, and in fact when I got a customised chair with a table attached, the situation was greatly improved. Meanwhile, however, the solution chosen was to make me a harness. I was duly measured up by one of the occupational therapists, and after a few days along she came with her construction – the ubiquitous Velcro very much in evidence. I was strapped in like a baby in a buggy. Cough or no cough, I was going nowhere!

Before very long, political considerations became evident. A wheelchair to go home in had to be provided for me by my own local authority. The hospital was associated with a different local authority, so there was a dispute over funding. Further complications arose because my local authority would not normally provide a chair unless the patient was actually going home. There was no immediate prospect of that. A lengthy spell of rehabilitation was the plan, and that not yet. So after much discussion, to which I was fortunately not privy, the wheelchair advisor for my home area agreed to provide me with a chair for use in the hospital and thereafter. She duly came to the hospital, accompanied by her technician, and bringing a 'suitable' wheelchair for me. It was quite an occasion, this first visit. All manner of interested persons gathered to have their say. There were physiotherapists, occupational therapists, members of the ward staff and, in his capacity as my advocate, Iain. The wheelchair advisor introduced herself and her technician to me, and explained as if to a simpleton why she was there. That was the only time anyone spoke directly to me. I was hoisted out of bed and into the 'new' chair. I still felt like a rag doll and considered that I was being pulled about as if I were one. The chair was attacked with spanners and screwdrivers. Parts of the chair and parts of me were rearranged 'to achieve a good position'. 'The Position' was discussed and evaluated by everyone assembled. I began to feel surplus to requirements. If only I could have said something, I would have nipped this insensitive (and ignorant) behaviour in the bud. But a terse, pithy comment was not an option so, after putting up with this for long enough, I started to cry. I was patted, told 'there, there' and they continued as before. This was like a red rag to a bull. Although completely unable to make a sound of my own volition, when I became very emotional I made noises. I began to wail. That, although childish and undignified, was the only thing I had at my disposal to make people take notice of me. Iain looked shocked. The others started to look uncomfortable.

"She is getting upset," someone said. Upset? I was furious! How dare they treat anyone like this, let alone an intelligent member of the same, or similar, profession? This was another example of the widespread attitude that if a person cannot talk, he or she is not capable of rational or intelligent thought. I have met this attitude many times during the course of my recovery. Often from people who should know better. The excuse that it is a sign of their own discomfiture or inadequacy is a lame one. These feelings of discomfiture are of little consequence when compared with the feeling of the intelligent mind trapped in a useless body.

The wheelchair advisor was escorted from the room, to allow me 'a rest'. The younger physiotherapist, who was looking increasingly uneasy by this stage, asked me if I would rather stop and continue another day.

"Get it over with," was my opinion. I did not want to encounter that woman on any more occasions than absolutely necessary. Of course, the precise nature of my thoughts could not be broadcast (perhaps fortunately) but I did get the message across that we should continue. The lady in question was ushered back in. She was rather subdued, and was careful to speak directly to me. She could not, however, remove the patronising tone in her voice when addressing me. I remained scornful of her lack of empathy.

I had cause to meet this lady several times during the early part of my recovery, as my wheelchair needs changed. Each encounter was extremely uncomfortable – on my part at least – but my recovery was spurred on by my determination to do the things which she professed I would be incapable of doing.

The nurse who was with me when I first moved my head played a major part in many of the milestones I passed in the early part of my recovery. It was she who cut and removed the temporary wires that held my gastrostomy tube until it was capable of staying in place just with the retaining balloon. I was thrilled and excited when she announced that the next day, given sufficient staff to help, I could have a real bath! This was a major undertaking. I was completely helpless, so had to be undressed, lifted onto a special, horizontal hoist and strapped in for safety. Covered up, I was then wheeled to the bathroom and lowered into the adjustable bath. The water had to be kept away from my tracheostomy, my head had to be supported, and the other various tubes about my person had to be accommodated. Despite all this palaver, it was bliss to have a bath after all this time. It was wonderful to feel the warm water lapping around my useless body, and after this 'proper' bath I felt so much cleaner than after the usual blanket bath. Family members would time their visits to coincide with bath time so that they could help out. This would release one nurse to other tasks, and it would make the likelihood of my having a 'proper' bath greater. Bath time was quite a business, but it was certainly worth it!

The spring sunshine was attracting many of the patients into the little garden attached to the back of the ward. One sunny day the senior nurse announced that I needed some sun and that she would wheel my bed outside. This seemed very daring, but I felt immensely grateful. Apart from anything else, it would be a change of scenery. But in fact the sunshine and fresh air were simply wonderful; I had had no idea just how much I had missed them. Going outside showed me the origins of some of the hallucinations which I suffered from in the early days. The 'ship's engine' noise was actually the air conditioning unit only a stone's throw away from the main building. The windows of the Intensive Care Unit overlooked the little garden. It felt so good to be able to orientate myself after all this time. To put the various places I had been, or was now, into context was a great help. At first I was taken outside in my bed, but as time went on, and I was encouraged to spend longer in the hospital wheelchair, I was pushed into the garden in that. I was also taken for 'walks' around the hospital, and later even to the local shops. Thus I gradually managed to put this new world into some sort of perspective.

Minuscule movements were beginning to return (a finger here, a toe there) and I became excited about each one. I have already described the delight as my eyes started to move from side to side (at first they would only move up and down). I then found to my great satisfaction that I could make myself go cross-eyed. This was fun! I had often pulled faces before the stroke and had earned the reputation of having a very expressive face. So with great glee I carried on 'practising' (or so I thought). After a while, though, I became very confused, as the two images I contrived to produce remained. I spent most of the day staring at the picture on the opposite wall. To my consternation this one picture became two. I could not make it go to a single image at all. I discovered later that although the muscles working my left eye were behaving correctly, those that would pull my right eye outwards were paralysed, and so it was pointing stubbornly in towards my nose. I was permanently boss-eyed. I was already reluctant to look at myself in the mirror (that, after all, is how I missed this happening). Now I really loathed what I saw. And everywhere I looked, there were two images. This double vision was to plague me for years afterwards.

As Iain was a doctor, the doctors looking after me were happy to share opinions and information with him. He, in turn, discussed everything with me. After he had been shown the angiograms of my brain, and seen the damage and its cause, it was agreed that if I wanted, I too should see them. I was curious, and not a little defiant. The euphoria of having survived, apparently against all odds, had not yet worn off. In addition, throughout this whole business I have felt a strange detachment. Part of me has watched with interest as each stage of this debilitating process has unfolded, and each small ability been regained. At first I was fascinated by what was happening to me. The full horror of it all was slower to become apparent. We seem to have a defence mechanism – the 'it will never happen to me' attitude. Even as the realisation dawned that it was indeed happening to me, I still retained an academic interest in what was going on. So I was quite keen to see for myself the pictorial evidence of this 'insult'. Elinor came with me to see the x-rays. She, of course, was interested from a medical point of view. She was about to become a medical student, and may never see this type of stroke again during her career. She also came for moral support and to 'translate' (Iain and the girls were by far the slickest at making sense of my 'eye-flash' language). The x-ray pictures showed a dismal story. There was the damaged artery where the clot had broken free. There too was the network of blood vessels supplying the base of the brain; duly blocked off just above where the clot had come to rest. All the brain tissue in the vicinity of those blood vessels would have been starved of oxygen, would be dying off, and would be replaced by scar tissue. No nerve impulses could pass through that scar tissue. What a depressing picture.

"What about collateral circulation?" I flashed hopefully, clutching at straws. Perhaps other blood vessels would come to the rescue and start supplying the starved brain tissue. Unlikely. Still defiant, I decided to ask the question that had been burning for so long.

"You expected me to die, didn't you?" I challenged. The doctor looked shifty, and was quiet for a minute, then, rather shamefaced, admitted that he had.

"But obviously someone up there was looking after you," he said. So it would seem.

Throughout the period following the stroke I received regular visits from the Director of the Rehabilitation Centre, or his deputy. They would keep me up-to-date on the likely date when I could start rehabilitation, would check on what progress (if any) I had made, and would give snippets of advice on how to make life easier. I was quite upset when one day the doctor suggested that I should have injections to stop the spasms which kept affecting me. These spasms made my limbs go rigid. They would cause the limbs to tense up or even move, with strength that was hard to believe, but of course completely without control. It was extremely difficult, and sometimes impossible, for the nurses to do anything with the limb in this condition, and for some people (though mercifully not for me) these spasms are very painful. They are thus regarded as 'not a good thing'. The injection of a toxin into the offending muscle would paralyse it and stop the unwanted movements. Imagine! As if I wasn't paralysed enough! Besides, I wanted any little improvement to be able to manifest itself, and not be masked by the work of this poison. So I refused. This was not a popular decision. But it was accepted. This was perhaps the first indication to the health professionals that I was not necessarily going to obey blindly. I had my own ideas for my recovery (such as it was) and I might just follow them.

My first outing after the stroke was while I was still in the hospital. I was still chairman of my local choral society, and the concert for which we were rehearsing when I had the stroke was coming up. I was wondering whether there was any chance of my being 'allowed out' when Iain suggested that very thing. I did not feel able to go to the actual performance – there were too many 'unknowns' about my condition and besides I had a tracheostomy, a gastrostomy and a urinary catheter, all of which would need looking after while we were out. Instead we agreed (and remember that I was still communicating by eye blinks) that it would be ideal for me to go to the dress rehearsal. A more informal occasion, we felt we could cope with all eventualities more easily, and I would still be supporting the society. The ward staff were all in favour of this enterprise; they were keen to plan what I should wear and what I would need to take with me on my jaunt. There were, however, quite a few logistical considerations to be dealt with. First, a vehicle. One that could transport me in the wheelchair. That could be hired from a local charity. Then the timing. Iain would be in the performance that evening. I was going to watch the afternoon's rehearsal. We had to fit a round trip of fifty miles in between rehearsal and performance. It could just be managed. I would need 'looking after' while Iain was otherwise engaged. A good friend was roped in to do that. She would also top up my gastrostomy. A big bottle of water and an oversized syringe were packed for that purpose. What would I wear? The ward staff seemed more excited and taxed by this question than I was. I gave Iain a list of what I wanted; clothes and makeup that I had not seen for months. Jewellery too; pieces of great sentimental value which I used to wear all the time and which had been removed at the start of my hospitalisation.

The day dawned. My clothes had arrived and Iain went to collect the vehicle. I was spruced up, dressed and made up. A look in the mirror revealed a complete stranger; one with a twisted face and an eye that turned in towards her nose. These were my clothes but they did not hang right; they had been arranged in position. Moreover, this stranger dribbled. A constant, glistening stream exuded from her mouth. This could not be me, could it? I did not want to know. I did not like what I saw, so I would not look. I allowed myself to be prepared for my outing. Then I was taken out to the 'van', fastened in safely for the journey, and off we set.

During the journey I was constantly surprised at the familiarity of the road and the landmarks en route. I still harboured the suspicion (hope?) that this was all a bad dream. To my consternation, all the signs suggested that it wasn't. This was for real, and there was no escape.

As we drew up in the car park our friends leapt up to take over my care, and we made our way into the concert venue. On the way in we met various members of the society and they each stopped and spoke to me, either expressing delight at my being there or giving me some words of encouragement. I burst into tears! This was not meant to happen. Speech was obviously out of the question, but I had thought that a gracious smile would be in order. It meant such a lot to me to see them. The society had been through a bad patch, but together we had weathered the storm and I believed that we had emerged relatively successfully. I had a huge sense of responsibility and even affection towards the members of the society, and I considered it very important that I should support them. But I had not reckoned with my lack of self-control. As each person came up to speak to me I burst into tears. With the tears, my arms and legs became extremely stiff and shot straight out in front of me. This caused severe distress to everyone who came to greet me, and it caused me great fury with myself. I was mortified at my 'bad behaviour', causing these well-meaning people such alarm. Worse, however, was to come.

Everyone settled down for the performance. I had rehearsed this with them. I knew this oratorio – almost off by heart. Now

I couldn't sing a note. Again I burst into tears and this time, emotions aroused, I wailed like a banshee. For someone who could not speak or otherwise use my vocal chords as I wanted I was certainly making a lot of noise. I fought like hell to get myself back under control – with only limited success. With dismay I remembered the article Iain had read to me about inappropriate, uncontrollable laughter and crying associated with stroke. I thought I could beat it. Obviously I could not.

Despite all this, the outing was deemed a success. All the practicalities worked. We could manage (albeit with help). We could do it again.

I was beginning to think that I could breathe quite well without my tracheostomy. I also wanted to start trying to talk. This was impossible with the type of tracheostomy tube I had. But before I could shed it, I had to pass two tests. Firstly I had to manage with the tube blocked off for two hours. The idea was to start with it blocked off for a short time, then build up to longer periods. This I duly did, and it wasn't long before I achieved this respiratory independence. I coughed a bit, and my body needed to put quite a bit of effort into inhalation at times, but on the whole I coped reasonably well. I was keen to move on to the second test. To block off the tube for twenty-four hours. This was a different matter altogether. The first few hours were fine. Thereafter, however, my breathing became laboured, and I coughed and coughed. I became quite distressed. The coughing started to make my throat bleed. Stubbornly I carried on. I wanted rid of this thing, and I would not be beaten! Then, towards the end of the twenty-four hours, I began to feel dreadful. Breathing was terribly difficult; I sucked in each breath with a huge effort and a terrifying, strangulated noise. I coughed up an alarming amount of blood. Then the world around me began to fade. Voices began to come and go. I was fighting, fighting. I realised that I was achieving nothing; I was just damaging myself. My stubbornness would not last the twenty-four hours. At least, it might, but I would not. So, with reluctance and yet relief, I gave up. The tube was unblocked, and I breathed again. I had failed.

We considered the situation carefully. We concluded that the tube itself was blocking my airway, and I would continue to have the same problem unless I had a smaller tube. Another benefit of having a doctor for a husband; Iain discussed the problem with the doctor, and it was decided to change the tube for a smaller one.

Although I did not relish the thought of a tube change (on the previous occasions there had been a lot of blood, a lot of coughing, and I had felt absolutely awful), the suggestion of a smaller, less intrusive tube was very welcome. Even better, I would be able to talk, or 'vocalise' as the therapists called it. I was eager to try talking. All kinds of technological wizardry, such as a **Light Writer** had been suggested, but I wanted to talk. Stubbornly, I wasn't interested in these substitutes for the real thing. However hard it was going to be (and I had no idea of just how hard), I was determined to persevere.

So, this time with a minimum of fuss, I had my tracheostomy tube replaced by what was in fact a child's one. My breathing was not adversely affected, and I seemed to cough much less. Blocking it off was just a matter of sticking some tape over it, and I could cope with it being blocked off so much better.

I hadn't realised what a complicated business speaking was. As the muscles of my face and jaw slackened a little, I felt that I should be able to start speaking again, but they remained paralysed and would not give the words their shape; my tongue lay limp and almost lifeless in my mouth. My vocal chords, severely weakened, needed a powerful breath behind them to make them vibrate. A power that I did not have. The soft palate too, plays an important part. So often taken for granted, out of sight, it must move up and down at the right times to divert the breath either up through the nose or out through the mouth, depending on the sound required. All this normally happens automatically, without thought. It no longer happened at all for me. If I wanted to talk again I would have to re-learn to make a sound and shape it into a word. Back to square one – and beyond! The visiting speech therapists were pleased because I was vocalising already. The involuntary grunts and moans that accompanied most of my exhalations were actually of some value! However I had to get them under control, as they were nothing but an embarrassment to me at that moment.

I delivered my first word to my daughters when they came in to see me.

"Hello," I greeted them, to their surprise and delight. Actually it sounded more like 'erro', but it was a start. From then on, I was keen to try out odd words on all and sundry. It was a triumph when I said 'morning' (or what passed for that) to my physiotherapists.

One morning, as usual, the nurse was changing the dressing around my tracheostomy. It was tied behind my neck and it was always a slightly worrying time when the ties were undone. As I was constantly warned: 'One good cough and the tube will be out'. I was always careful to breathe as smoothly as I could, and not to do anything to provoke a cough. This was just a normal day, and I lay quiet and still for my dressing to be changed. The ties were undone. The nurse turned away to prepare something. I swallowed. I didn't cough or feel anything untoward. But when the nurse turned back towards me, the tracheostomy tube lay on the pillow. It was out! I was delighted. The nurse was appalled. She went off to phone a higher authority to see what she should do. Meanwhile, I felt fine. I could breathe quite easily, and had no pain. Besides, I had been trying to get rid of the thing for weeks – I wasn't about to allow it back in! True, it had probably contributed to keeping me alive in the early days, but it was uncomfortable, it made me cough, stopped me talking (or so I perceived) and I hated it. I was very relieved when the nurse returned saying it could stay out. She covered the hole in my neck with a dressing.

One tube out, two to go! I felt that I was getting somewhere.

9. Rehabilitation begins

At the beginning of June it was announced that there was a place ready for me at the local rehabilitation centre. There had been promises of a date for my transfer for some time, but owing to various problems with staffing levels this had repeatedly been deferred. This time, however, everything seemed to be in order and arrangements were made for me to go to the unit. It was now eleven weeks since the stroke.

I was fortunate in that this was arguably one of the best neurological rehabilitation units in the country. I had frequently been told that 'you will be all right when you get to Brookfield' (this is not its real name) and that 'things will be so much better when you get to Brookfield'. I couldn't see how they would be able to work miracles. Yet my expectations were still very high. I left the ward vowing to 'work hard' with the firm belief that with time and hard work I would regain most of my previous ability.

I also left with several promises of visits. Along the way I had become quite fond of several members of staff, and it was not easy to say goodbye to them.

Moving day dawned. I was very glad that Iain would accompany me; I was inordinately thankful to have him by my side whenever I had to face anything unpleasant or new. He was even going to spend the night with me. Under these circumstances I felt that I could cope. No matter that I could neither move nor speak. Iain would do the talking for me, and ensure that my physical needs were attended to.

I took with me my leg splints, arm splints and 'T-roll' (a large, firm cushion shaped like the letter 'T', which was used to keep my legs and hips bent and knees apart). The splints were always used at night time. I looked not unlike a mummy – it was hardly an elegant way to go to sleep!

I seemed to have so many goodbyes to say. I was touched

that quite a number of people made a special visit to the ward to wish me well. A few even promised to come and see how I was getting on. I wondered how many I would see again.

The ambulance took me to the other side of the city. How many times had I passed that way and been completely unaware that the place existed? Totally hidden from the road, and down a fairly long, winding drive, we came across the collection of long, low buildings that was the rehabilitation centre.

I was taken inside the 'ward' (the living accommodation – the other buildings were therapy areas) and introduced to my 'primary nurse' – the nurse who took overall responsibility for me during my stay at the rehabilitation centre. There were two teams of nurses; each patient was allocated to one of these teams, and within that team to a particular nurse. My 'team' provided the majority of my care; in this way each person would know and be known tolerably well by a group of others. Over the next few days I met the various members of 'my team' and I got to know them and they me during the ensuing weeks and months. I was given a tour around and the set up was explained.

We were each given a weekly timetable, tailored to our individual needs. It comprised forty-minute periods (not unlike school) of each of the following subjects: physiotherapy, speech and language therapy, occupational therapy (including what to do with leisure time) and psychotherapy (perhaps to help us come to terms with what had happened). I needed all the therapies! My timetable was full. There were free periods. These were for rest, and visitors were encouraged to wait until the working day was over to drop in, as the schedule was felt to be too full and important to be interrupted.

The patients undergoing rehabilitation could be divided into two main groups, although everyone had had some kind of 'insult' to their brain. There were people who had sustained head injuries in accidents, and there were those who had had strokes of various kinds and varying degrees of severity. There were also a few who had suffered a brain disease of some kind; these were outnumbered by the two main groups. Many of those with head injuries following an accident had changed personalities, impaired intellect, and many couldn't speak. Generally, those who had suffered strokes had weakness or paralysis in one or more limbs, and some had difficulty in finding the right word when talking (dysphasia). But nearly all of them <u>could</u> talk, and despite some having minor character changes, they were not disruptive and their basic intelligence was not in question. I was by far the most physically affected stroke patient there. I was completely paralysed, couldn't eat or drink properly, and couldn't talk. I seemed to some to have more in common with the most seriously brain-damaged patients. But my intellectual capacity was undiminished. My memory, my judgement, my ability to calculate were all intact. So I noticed when people talked down to me. I became angry when some members of staff were patronising in their attitudes to me; incensed when the younger staff were disrespectful. I watched, critically, as the other patients were attended to, making judgements about the attitudes and even the competence of staff members. I quickly decided whom I trusted and whom I did not.

My intact intellect in the face of so much physical disability caused problems for some members of staff.

"They haven't ever met anyone like you," excused the Nurse-in-Charge after a particularly patronising episode, during which I had managed to show my displeasure fairly effectively. *Tough*, thought I, *I'm not stupid, and I refuse to allow myself to be treated as if I am.* Throughout this whole business I have been very sensitive about the way people treat me. Towards the end of my time in the hospital I had begun to feel like a quirky pet. Some members of staff would greet me perfunctorily as they entered or left the ward, much as one might make conversation with the dog, or perhaps a hamster in a cage. They didn't expect a reply, and of course they got none. But how I wished I could surprise them with a terse, vaguely sarcastic retort. To this day I get very angry at the merest hint of being patronised; sensitive perhaps, but I do still expect a modicum of respect.

During the first couple of days I was introduced to my therapists. My speech therapist was an attractive, cheerful young mum, recently returned from maternity leave after the birth of her first child. She was assigned the task of finding out my expectations of rehabilitation and any strengths I possessed that might help me attain the goals I set myself. The physiotherapist was a big girl who seemed to attract (or be lumbered with) the 'difficult'

– i.e. the violent or downright unpleasant – patients. She certainly didn't show any nervousness in dealing with them; she had a very assertive, even brash, manner which I assume was intended to engender respect. She professed the belief that we would get along really well. In fact our personalities clashed before much time had elapsed, and thereafter our relationship – although not unpleasant – was somewhat strained. My occupational therapist was a pleasant, smiling girl, who was eager to find me some enjoyable way of passing the time. She asked what hobbies I had enjoyed before the stroke, and was dismayed to be told that they included playing the piano, cookery, yoga and needlework. All needing active arms and legs and good eyesight. Her task would have been so much easier had I been a couch potato! She offered me the use of some 'environmental controls'. I was still reluctant to accept technological help, believing that with hard work my physical faculties would be coaxed back into action, but I agreed – thinking that after all it would only be a temporary measure. So I was provided with a television, a video recorder, a radio and a tape recorder. There was a control box with a switch. The movement in my head and neck had improved enough for me to manage to control the switch by turning my head. The alarm was connected, as were a light and a fan, so by pressing the switch when the required item was illuminated I could use all these things myself. In these small areas I was no longer dependent on others.

This OT left after a few weeks, and was replaced by a very bright girl. She seemed to see my difficulties as a challenge, and tried to find a practical solution to each problem put in front of her.

The last therapist I had to meet was my psychologist. Sessions with him were meant for discussion of difficulties, fears for the future, grief for the life left behind, and so on. I still had a very positive attitude. I was convinced that with a lot of hard work I could return to 'normality'; that this was only temporary. I was fascinated by what was going on. As a student of psychology I found the changing relationships around me, and the effect the situation was having on everyone, a source of great interest. As a wife, a mother, and an intelligent woman, now paralysed and mute, I was devastated. I tended to avoid the long term issues, believing that they would cease to be relevant. I stuck to the immediate hurt; how members of my family were coping, my dislike of so many people's patronising attitude and so on. Discussions were of course impossible. I found this extremely frustrating as I find a good discussion very rewarding. I had three psychologists during my time in rehabilitation (there was at that time quite a high turnover of psychology staff) and they all approached me with varying degrees of apprehension. My lack of effective language made me seem as alien as if I had grown two heads. Though, to give them their due, all three began by stating that they would find out what I wanted to say, whatever it took. Only the second of the three seemed to have a real insight into how I felt. She could do a mean impression of a patronising attitude, and volunteered an accurate description of what I would like to do to anyone displaying one!

She didn't baulk at discussing the possibility of my seeking suicide. I felt quite lost when she went on maternity leave.

The first couple of weeks were set aside for assessment – to see what I could and couldn't do. I could do very little. The difference in the attitudes of the various therapists was very marked. In physiotherapy I felt a complete failure. It was as if I was given a challenge, and there was great disappointment in my inability to meet it. I was delighted, however, at any small movement which returned. Quite often it was the 'wrong kind of movement' and I was urged not to practise it. Imagine my frustration; I wanted to push my body really hard, to make it move again. I felt sure that with a positive mental attitude and relentless effort I could make some impression on the paralysis. Instead I felt like a 'no-hoper', and was encouraged to accept my lot. I felt like the living example of a page in a textbook; the page that deals with rare and severe conditions that have no real prospect of improvement. I felt, and continue to feel, a mix of desperate sadness and downright anger. How <u>dare</u> they write me off?

My speech therapist, however, seemed to be much more open-minded, with a 'see-how-it-goes' type attitude. She put a high priority on my being able to communicate – by whatever method – with the maximum number of people. I could not use the usual alphabet charts as my eyes would not move around the letters on the chart. I had to continue with my 'eye flashes'. She therefore discussed with the family how we had developed our system of communication and the best way of using it. They acknowledged my wish to get my speech back, and a system of trying to speak words, or spelling them out when speaking whole words was unsuccessful, was devised. If that failed I would revert to the eye flashes.

As time went on, and either my speech improved or staff became attuned to my efforts, less of our communication was made using eye flashes and more through speech. I did feel that I had failed if I had to spell out a word in eye flashes and I would get very cross when that happened. I got a severe talking to from my speech therapist. It was the communication that mattered, not the method. I was partly chastened.

The staff held meetings, run by my speech therapist, on 'how to communicate with Margaret'. There was no escaping the fact that I was different: from other people, other stroke patients. I felt very uncomfortable. It wasn't anyone's fault; that's just the way it was!

As well as communication, my speech therapist was also responsible for improving my swallowing. She made an assessment of it early on. The swallowing mechanism wasn't working properly. Another function that we all take for granted. Until it goes wrong. I started taking a great interest in what is involved in swallowing, asking exactly what movements are involved so that I could concentrate on each one. I was sent for a 'video fluoroscopy'. I had to swallow differing thicknesses of liquid while my swallowing mechanism was watched on an x-ray video. I was dismayed to be told that with all but the thickest liquid some had trickled down towards my lungs. I was not closing off my airway, so there was the constant danger that I might choke. Great caution had to be exercised with my food and drink, and this was policed by the speech therapists.

It also fell to my speech therapist to complete the form which all patients had to fill in before embarking on rehabilitation. Everybody had to state their aims for rehabilitation, and their expectation of how long it would take. I intended to be up and walking (maybe with help) and able to use my arms and hands, perhaps not as well as before, but well enough to get by. With some trepidation she asked me how long I expected to be in the rehabilitation unit. She was visibly relieved when I 'said' a year. Some people, she replied, expected results overnight. I was prepared for a long, hard haul. But I did not consider not succeeding. Neither did I consider being unable to talk properly. Life without language was inconceivable. There were people who seemed to think that I should embrace alternative methods of communication, but I rejected these; however hard it was going to prove to be, I intended to learn to speak again. I was asked what quality I possessed which I considered would best help my rehabilitation. 'Bloody-mindedness' was my response. A little taken aback, my speech therapist laughed nonetheless. And it has indeed proved thus. There have been many times when only sheer belligerence has kept me going. It has sometimes presented those who look after me with a challenge or has even infuriated them, but I consider that a small price to pay for my survival.

My physiotherapist greeted my aims with dismay. She preferred to set much lower goals (or so it seemed to me). These included, 'to be independent in a powered wheelchair'. I did not like the sound of that. Although paralysed, pushed about in a chair and dumb, I honestly considered my situation to be purely temporary. Anything else was inconceivable. I felt ready to rise to the challenge, and felt bitterly disappointed at what I considered was my physiotherapist's defeatist attitude.

There was one last group of therapists I had to meet, and that was the occupational therapists running the 'leisure' activities. It seemed their intention was to teach or develop someone's existing skills to fill their free time. These would exercise weak limbs, or retrain a body with limited movement, and at the same time provide useful occupation and even enjoyment to a victim of brain injury. I obviously presented them with a problem. None of my limbs worked, and my interests were not of the 'couch potato' variety. I took an almost instant dislike to the set-up because the young therapist in charge talked to me in the childish, singsong voice so often reserved for the dim-witted. She had decided that I should try silk painting. No great accuracy was needed to produce an acceptable design and the minimum effort gave maximum effect. It was suggested that I hold the paintbrush in my mouth. My hands did not move but my head did. Hold the brush between my teeth and move my head. Problem solved! I complied. I didn't like it however. I did not want to paint with my mouth. It would be admitting defeat I thought.

The therapist had another bright idea. She brought out a contraption which she strapped to my head. The brush fitted in the front of it, and as I moved my head, the brush moved along the silk. I liked that even less. I felt thoroughly miserable. Without dignity, or respect. Without hope. From then on I did my utmost to avoid these sessions. Like a naughty school kid I played truant, finding all manner of excuses not to go: I 'felt too tired' or 'was expecting a visitor'.

One other thing that had to be done in the first week or so was an eye check. My eyesight was pretty dreadful; the main problem being the double vision. I had had excellent eyesight before the stroke (I had always felt rather smug about that) so I was very intolerant of this added complication. With my inability to speak or move, it was very difficult for the orthoptist to test my eyes. But she persisted, and in the end came up with the suggestion that I could try wearing a patch over one eye. She duly produced a selection of sticky patches ('adhesive occluders') and stuck one over my immobile eye. It did solve the double vision, but made my face itch. I also thought I must look like a casualty from the battle-front! Yet more sucking of teeth by the therapist accompanied this assessment of my vision. It seemed that my eyesight was doomed as well as the rest of me. Did I have nothing functional left?

Iain had spent the first night with me. He sat at my bedside, dozing when he was able to and holding my hand. I learned later that this unnerved the night staff, and earned him the description of my 'Rottweiler'. I learned this much later, when we had become friendly with some of the staff, and we were able to joke about it. The following day Iain was cornered by the nurse in charge who made him promise that he would not spend the night sitting in a chair by my side again. He was to collect an empty bed, make it up, and spend the night sleeping comfortably in my room. He didn't argue. This was better than we could ever have hoped for. From then on, one night per week, Iain would stay with me. We would spend the evening watching television or doing something ordinary and domestic, then at bedtime we would snuggle down together (almost), just like at home. I had wondered so often whether I would ever sleep with my husband again. The future was one step closer to being less bleak. I had something to look forward to. The significance of our spending the night together on a regular basis cannot be overestimated.

10. Food, glorious food

Food has always played an immensely important part in my life. I loved preparing it, and spent hours poring over cookery books and magazines, selecting recipes. Nothing gave me greater pleasure than seeing family and friends gathered around our table, eating and chatting. I fancied myself as a good cook and a relaxed hostess. Of late Iain and I had had some success with growing and making our own fresh produce, and it was a great treat for us to have an excellent meal out. This fondness for all things culinary resulted in me having a constant battle with my weight – of fluctuating severity. However, at the time of my stroke I was reasonably slim.

For several months, food was absent from my life. Food that we would recognise as such, that is. For the first few months I was tube-fed. Early on, in the intensive care unit, I was visited by a dietician who, from my height and weight, calculated the number of calories I would need daily. This was translated into the number of bottles of special liquid feed I would need, plus a carefully calculated amount of water. To begin with I was fed through a nasogastric tube, then after several weeks (by which time I had been moved to the main neurological ward) I was fitted with the gastrostomy tube. The 'food' and water were delivered direct to my stomach, the rate controlled by an electric pump. Eating and drinking were out of the question. My facial and mouth muscles were paralysed, I had great difficulty swallowing, and my jaws were clamped shut. Shut, that is, until I yawned, coughed, or did anything that involved involuntarily opening my mouth. I have previously described the effects of my jaws crashing down on my tongue or cheeks if they got in the way of my teeth. They met with tremendous pressure, and continued to bite down hard. Very soon I had a chewed and extremely sore mouth. Over time I became able to keep my cheeks and tongue free of my cruel teeth, and between these yawning episodes my mouth remained resolutely shut. Keeping my mouth clean and feeling fresh was both important and difficult. The miniature sponges used for care of the mouth had to be squeezed through my closed lips and manoeuvred as effectively as possible inside my cheeks. Getting at the centre of my mouth was just impossible.

Being tube fed, and therefore having substances deposited straight into my stomach, meant that I avoided tasting things. This was a definite advantage in the case of the liquid feed. It smelled vile, and on the unfortunate (but mercifully rare) occasions that I burped and regurgitated a little, tasted even worse. When the intravenous drips had been removed, most of the drugs I required could, in their liquid forms, be administered through my tube. So I didn't object to any unpleasant-tasting medicine – I hardly noticed it. The one exception to this was heparin – a blood-thinning drug – which had to be injected daily. My abdomen was chosen as the site for this. I disliked having any kind of injection and had never had one into my abdomen before. I used to dread the daily puncture, and I also dreaded the daily blood test which preceded it.

However, the injections would continue until the results of this blood test were satisfactory, and then the drug would be changed to one which could be put down my gastrostomy tube. The number of days that this continued seemed interminable, and my tummy got very sore. But I was becoming accustomed to undergoing uncomfortable, unpleasant and even painful procedures. This was just another to add to the list.

I longed for the taste of something sharp and refreshing in my mouth. I craved a drink of grapefruit juice – my usual breakfast drink. But I couldn't open my mouth. Even if I could have done, my swallowing was haphazard and unreliable. There was every chance that any liquid I swallowed would end up not in my stomach, but in my lungs. One of us came up with the idea of putting some juice in a syringe and sliding the syringe into my mouth between my cheek and gums. The juice could then be squeezed into my mouth and I could swallow it. The syringe came from Iain's medical bag and we washed it after use and kept it hidden in my drawer ready for the next time.

This was highly unorthodox, even dangerous, so we kept it secret from the staff to begin with. I did not want to be stopped. Particularly when my sister started bringing me little bottles of ready-mixed gin and tonic to put in my syringe. It was lovely to have a refreshing taste in my mouth, and as for the gin and tonic – that was a real treat! I had a feeling of conspiratorial delight when my sister came to visit and delved into her bag to bring out a small bottle of clear, innocuous-looking liquid.

The medical staff were so concerned that my jaw continued to remain clamped shut that they wanted to inject the jaw with botulinum toxin. The idea was to weaken the strong muscles which closed my jaw, thus allowing my mouth to open. I resisted this vehemently. Nowadays people pay vast amounts of money to have their facial wrinkles smoothed out by botox injections into their facial muscles, and many people suffering from agonising muscle-spasms have derived great benefit from it. But I didn't want this poison, however much diluted, in my body. In addition, my reasoning was that my body was paralysed enough as it was. I had no intention of introducing more paralysis. So, rightly or wrongly, wisely or foolishly, I stubbornly refused this treatment, much to the exasperation of my doctors.

Then, just as their frustration became palpable, my mouth began to open! The tension in my jaws began to slacken, and I was able to part my teeth and lips a few millimetres. I felt triumphant.

Now I had to try to exercise my lips and tongue. I was exhorted to make odd shapes with my mouth, to lick as many envelopes and stamps as possible. Both were a tall order, as my lips were like wood and my tongue refused to protrude. It stayed resolutely in my mouth. It could have been a beached whale, wallowing in the shallows – it just lay there, doing nothing.

I was visited by members of the hospital speech therapy team. One lady specialised in communication – non-verbal and verbal. She came armed with a boxful of charts and gadgets; most were useless to me as they needed good eyesight or agile hands and I had neither. Another therapist specialised in speech. She gave me exercises to get my mouth moving; a task as difficult for me as giving a double-decker bus a push-start on an uphill slope. Yet another favoured trying out different foods to see which I could manage best. Finally there was the lady whose specialty was swallowing. She was horrified that I was drinking 'straight' fruit juice (I kept quiet about the gin and tonic!). Tactfully she pointed out that for swallowing safety, fluids should be thickened (with a proprietary, supposedly tasteless powder). Meanwhile she suggested that I should start with something the consistency of yoghurt, taken off a spoon.

Iain or the girls used to spend the whole day with me, and they would bring themselves a packed lunch which they ate at my bedside. What delights lurked inside those plastic picnic boxes! Sandwich fillings which I would have previously considered either mundane or outrageous became tantalising. The look of pained resignation with which I watched my family tuck in caused much amusement and not a little sheepishness on their part. Even hospital food became attractive. I was tormented by the tempting smells emanating from the trolleys which regularly arrived on the ward. I craved a plate of chips, a good stew; even boiled fish would have been acceptable. But I was stuck with my fruit yoghurt – or chocolate mousse, which is what I preferred. I couldn't have eaten any of the things I craved, even if no-one had forbidden them. My facial muscles weren't up to biting or chewing. My tongue could not toss the food around my mouth, and I found swallowing so difficult that apart from the danger of the food going into my lungs instead of my stomach I could not guarantee getting anything down anyway. So chocolate mousse it was! Iain would come armed with the pot of it and a teaspoon for my daily 'eating practice'. I had no idea what a complicated business eating is. It is one of the many functions of daily life that we all take for granted. I was affronted that it was no longer an automatic process.

My first attempts at eating were calamitous. There has to be some synchronisation between breathing and swallowing. In addition, if one needs to exhale when one's mouth is full, one does so through the nose. I had not mastered either of these, and to make matters worse, I was prone to involuntary deep breaths (with consequent forceful exhalations). So with every mouthful there was the likelihood of my spitting chocolate mousse – sometimes over large distances, and certainly over me or Iain. I still had a tracheostomy and frequently coughed uncontrollably. I was said to have an 'incomplete swallow', so every time I swallowed there was a real danger of food (and even saliva) heading down my trachea into my lungs, as well as down the oesophagus into my stomach. Everyone has a reflex to cope with this eventuality; a good cough usually sends things in the right direction and anything getting stuck provokes a fit of choking. My cough reflex was undamaged and strong so this regularly propelled chocolate mousse over long distances. Many people said that being able to cough so forcefully was a good thing; I could 'always protect my airway'. This is undoubtedly true, but as someone who was brought up always to cover their mouth when they coughed (and who had instilled the same discipline into their children), being unable move my hand up to shield my mouth was extremely distressing. At first it could take twenty minutes to eat half a pot of mousse. The girls took their turn at feeding me, and with remarkable forbearance they and Iain would give me 'eating practice' every day. They endured chocolate spray in their faces, down their clothes, and all over their hands and arms as I spat, coughed, choked and dribbled my way through the pot. They endured it stoically, even cheerfully. I was ashamed. This was disgusting. Not for the first time I was behaving in a way that was a complete anathema to me. Was there to be no end to the ignominy I felt? Despite this, I was determined to eat again, and so we persevered. Eventually I felt that I could tackle food from the hospital menu. I was given the go-ahead and, apart from some general guidance from the speech therapist to choose soft food, I was left to my own devices. As I couldn't move, I had to be fed, and someone had to fill in my menu card for me. Quite often this was forgotten, so I got inappropriate food or none at all. Other times, although I had chosen the softest thing on the menu (such as spaghetti hoops), I found that I couldn't easily eat them. On many occasions when I was being fed by one of the nurses I would become so embarrassed by the mess I was making that I would only attempt a few mouthfuls. It was a good thing that I was still receiving my nourishment through my gastrostomy tube. Nothing that passed my lips could at this time be construed as a meal.

I was bemoaning all this (plus the fact that I was fed up

with the regular servings of cauliflower cheese) to a very good friend, who visited me regularly. She said she would see what she could do. So began my supply of tasty and tempting treats. I had no need of hospital food now. I tended to order something vaguely suitable for lunch from the hospital menu, and I didn't mind whether or not there was a nurse or anyone available to feed it to me. Because come supper time I had the choice of the delicacies which my friend had brought in, and which we kept, with permission, in the ward fridge. There was always a member of my family with me around that time to feed me; even my mother was roped in when she was visiting. I don't think I was any less messy then than I was when she used to feed me over forty years before!

I was very sensitive about the amount of mess I made. There was always a large pile of used tissues at the end of every 'meal'. This would attract thoughtless comments from various members of staff, who appeared to find the whole business very amusing. I joined in with their laughter. But inside I was squirming with embarrassment. I found the mess I made, and the coughing and spitting that I did, very hard to take.

The speech therapists were keen to investigate how good my swallowing was. Their way of testing this was to feed me natural yoghurt, coloured blue (yes, blue). Then, almost straight away, suction was carried out through my tracheostomy tube and the resulting substances examined. If there was any blue to be seen it would indicate that some food was sneaking down my airway and that my swallow was 'incomplete'– i.e. not safe. I dreaded the appearance of any blue colour in the suction tube. I desperately wanted to prove that I could swallow properly. But I was thwarted. A little blue continued to appear in the suction tube. Never a large amount, but sufficient to make the speech therapists plead caution. I was urged to eat only a small amount of creamy-textured food, and no liquid. Meanwhile the tube feeding of whitish liquid food and large quantities of water continued. I felt frustrated. This was admitting defeat, I thought. Recklessly, and secretly, I continued to quaff small amounts of gin and tonic and I began to suck chocolate buttons.

When I moved to the rehabilitation unit a more formal feeding regime was devised. I was allowed pureed food, and drinks which were thickened with special tasteless (well, theoretically) thickening powder.

The speech therapists here were equally concerned about whether or not I was swallowing properly, and persuaded me to undergo 'video fluoroscopy'. This entailed swallowing (either from a spoon or a paper cup) a quantity of barium-like fluid, flavoured with milkshake powder. The radio-opaque liquid could then be 'followed' by a real-time x-ray video, on its journey from the mouth to the stomach. The swallow is a complex mechanism involving muscles of the tongue, the throat and the oesophagus. The intricacies of this mechanism could be scrutinised by means of this moving x-ray. It was feared that some of the liquid would escape and go into my lungs, so I was fed a little from a teaspoon. The first liquid was fairly runny; the consistency of a normal drink. I determined not to cough and let myself down. To my intense irritation I coughed and spluttered, and the lady-in-charge announced (was it triumphantly?) that a significant amount of the liquid had headed for my lungs, and so that consistency of liquid was unsafe for me to drink. The video was repeated several times, with me being given progressively thicker versions of this non-too-pleasant liquid. When its consistency was such that it could only be spooned out of the cup (and not poured), it was deemed 'safe' – according to the pictures – for me to drink.

From then on, anything I wanted to drink had to be thickened with the special thickening powder and fed to me from a spoon. 'Solid' food was less of a problem; pureed was the correct consistency. The novelty of being given a 'meal', though, soon wore off. The food for me was plated-up at a central kitchen, several miles away. When it arrived it was, at best, three mounds of indeterminate grey or brown matter and, at worst, a hard, congealed mess. I soon started refusing to eat it, relying instead on the delicious food parcels from my friend and the luxury yoghurts brought in by my family. The nursing staff took pity on me and persuaded the swallowing expert that it was equally acceptable to give me the same food as 'normal' patients, freshly pureed in the unit kitchen. This was infinitely preferable; the food was vaguely recognisable. I was offered a greater variety and it was altogether more palatable.

I craved 'normal' food. What I would have given for a chip!

At supper time the other patients had sandwiches. Sandwiches in cellophane packets. Sandwiches with such fillings as chicken salad, prawn and mayonnaise, cheese and tomato. Never before had such things been so attractive. But they were not for me. I wasn't allowed them. I couldn't chew them, couldn't manage the crusts. They were probably right. In fact I had a much tastier alternative: one of the purees devised by my friend (e.g. guacamole, smoked salmon mousse or spicy summer vegetables) followed by one of the rich yoghurts or chocolate mousses brought in by my family.

It seemed that I was constantly receiving dire warnings of the consequences of trying to eat unsuitable food. Choking was predicted and aspiration pneumonia threatened. 'Dangerous' foods were expressly forbidden. I felt like a recalcitrant toddler. This was reinforced by the fact that I had to be fed. My different-ness was highlighted by the fact that none of the other patients could understand what I said (when I did venture to say anything), so I never built up a rapport with anyone. I have to admit that I was soon behaving like a recalcitrant toddler. I was constantly pushing at the boundaries, particularly where food was concerned, and I had the same sort of difficulties with communication – with similar consequences. To say that I was frustrated would be to understate wildly my predicament. I wasn't allowed to eat many of the foods I wanted to eat. I couldn't physically have managed them even if I had been. I was treated at best as a mischievous youngster and at worst as an unintelligent individual who could be placated, patronised and pitied. I fumed!

All this time, I was still being tube fed at night. The tube in my stomach was connected up to the electric pump at bedtime, and I received my daily quota of calories and fluid while I (supposedly) slept. So any food I took orally was an 'extra', and as I became more able to eat and drink, I received up to twice the amount of 'food' I required. The dietician was very reluctant to allow the tube feeding to be discontinued. She was concerned that it might not possible for me to take sufficient calories and (more importantly) fluid by mouth. I wanted to be rid of another tube. As it happened, I soon got my way, but in a completely unplanned and unprepared-for incident.

The gastrostomy tube was held in place by a small, water

filled balloon. The amount of water was checked and, if necessary, replenished weekly. It would be a disaster, I was told, if the tube should come out. It had to be replaced within half an hour, or else the hole and the path to my stomach would close up and replacement would be impossible. Because of this, and because mine had been a new and unusual procedure, a spare tube was kept locked in the cupboard of whichever ward I inhabited, 'just in case'.

By the time I had been transferred to the rehabilitation unit some weeks later all this had been forgotten. One morning, when I was being dried after a shower, the nurse rubbed a little vigorously and out popped my gastrostomy tube. It was quite painless; suddenly the tube was lying there in the towel. I was delighted! The nurse was not. This was a disaster. The tube would have to be replaced. But first the doctor had to be contacted. And they would have to get another tube. From another hospital. Because despite all the care that had previously been taken in the hospital to keep a spare tube close by, the rehabilitation unit did not have one. I was gleeful! It would take too long to get hold of a tube, plus find a doctor to fit it. The hole would have closed. I could be rid of another tube.

"Couldn't I do without it now?" I asked one of the nurses who understood my primitive speech reasonably well. After consultation with the dietician, she gave me my answer. No. The tube feeding had to continue. They couldn't be sure yet that I was taking sufficient calories or fluid orally. I tried to explain that there was a time pressure to this and that the hole would close, but my account fell on deaf ears. The young doctor was particularly dismissive. She couldn't understand much of what I said, and when she did understand my words she failed to understand my meaning. I felt (not for the first, or the last, time) that I was being humoured, but otherwise disregarded.

At last a replacement tube arrived and preparations were made. The half-hour deadline was well past. I was certain that the new tube would not go in. Inwardly I shrugged. Let them find out, I thought indignantly. They will perhaps discover that I do know a thing or two. Behind my feeling of defiance, I did worry slightly that attempting to pass a tube where it wouldn't go might hurt me. But I was still confident that I would be proved right.

Everything was prepared for fitting the new tube. A nurse wheeled in the necessary equipment and the doctor, hands scrubbed clean, swabbed my abdomen, opened the packet and tried to insert the tube. But it would not go in! Despite all the pushing and shoving, it would not budge. I was jubilant. The track into my stomach had closed up. Not only had I been proved right, but no longer would I have to endure those foul-smelling tube feeds, or that irritating 'tick, tick' sound of the pump beside my bed. I could eat real food (albeit pulverised) and real drinks (although thickened). This was progress.

The staff were not happy. I was given a lecture on getting sufficient calories and, more importantly, fluid into my system, or back to the gastrostomy it would be. I didn't see any problem in getting sufficient calories into my system, even if it did mean eating mush for a while. Besides, I had waited for this moment for months. I had no qualms about returning to 'normal' food and drink.

Mealtimes resembled a battlefield. To my chagrin, and acute embarrassment, I was unable to behave with anything like the decorum I deemed appropriate. I expected to be able to eat without thinking; it had always been an automatic process. But I still coughed and spat and dribbled. I was mortified. But I covered my embarrassment by laughing; my mess at meal-times was treated as a huge joke. I had to be fed, and while I was having pureed food, fed with a spoon. I had a bib put around my neck. I felt like a baby; and I felt I was treated like a child: 'You can't have this', 'You aren't allowed that'. How I hated that! Yet I played along. I laughed. I acted the lovable but mischievous youngster. For two reasons. Firstly, I couldn't come out with the quick ripostes which I thought were warranted. Then secondly, something in my upbringing dictated that I accept things graciously and politely. I tried to stay good humoured whatever.

However, one day I flipped. It was teatime. A member of staff made a flippant and dismissive remark to me in front of the other patients, all assembled for their meals. I was angry. But I felt powerless. I couldn't speak well enough to protest. I couldn't move quickly enough in my chair to make a theatrical exit. I burst into tears. It was all I could do – although I didn't contrive it. The nurses were appalled. I had never reacted in that way before. They didn't know what to do. They chided and scolded, cooed and fussed. But I was inconsolable. Weeks, months of pent-up anger and frustration came tumbling out. Found the only outlet left to me. The more the nurses beseeched me to stop crying, the more I bawled. They just didn't know what to do. They described me as 'distressed', 'overwrought', 'inconsolable'. I was just plain <u>angry</u>. They decided to send for Iain. He 'would be able to do something' with me. Iain was at a conference, some distance away. Ordinarily I wouldn't have dreamed of disturbing him. Or of suggesting that he should drive so far at that time of night. But this time I didn't protest. This time I would be consciously selfish. I wanted to see Iain. He would listen to me. He would understand.

So I was taken to my room to await Iain's arrival. At the same time it was announced that I had a visitor. My dread at being seen in such a state dissolved into relief and delight as I realised that my visitor was my brother-in-law. More like a brother to me, he too would listen to me. He could lighten my mood; could make me smile, or even laugh. He did all of that, and when Iain arrived I was considerably more relaxed. The nurses were visibly relieved to see Iain arrive. They could pass on the 'problem' to him. I felt relieved too. After the three of us had spent some time pleasantly chatting, my brother-in-law went home, leaving Iain and me to spend the night together. I was immensely glad to have Iain by my side, and I felt at peace with the world once more.

Feeding someone is a skilled task, a skill frequently underestimated. So often it is a job allocated to the most junior nurse, or the least familiar with the workings of a particular ward or the people on it. All too often it is seen as 'easy', 'undemanding', 'effortless' and unskilled. In fact it is a grave responsibility and a much more skilled task than is appreciated. I didn't realise this until I was on the receiving end of it. How vulnerable we are when we are unable to feed ourselves! Apart from the impossibility of sneaking the odd chocolate or biscuit, or getting a drink at will, we are dependent on someone else to give us the food we like in a manner which we find acceptable.

I quickly became very fussy. Not about the food itself (for I ate some peculiar-looking stuff, at some strange temperatures, and was glad of it), but about the way I was fed. Feeding someone well involves teamwork; it helps if each knows the other's foibles. Successful feeding is a matter of timing, of putting an acceptable amount on the spoon or fork, of putting the spoon or fork just the right distance into the mouth. It does require some empathy with the recipient. I would get very irritated with people who would tentatively poke food through my lips, causing me to strain to take hold of a meagre amount. Others annoyed me by obviously being more interested in the goings on around than they were in feeding me. I also got very agitated with those who thrust cleaning paper in my face while I was trying to chew my food (a messy face did upset me, but that upset me more). I have to confess that I wasn't easy to feed. I couldn't open my mouth wide – my jaws had, after all, been clamped tight shut for a long time and were still very stiff. In addition I coughed a great deal – and of course I couldn't cover my mouth, so I tended to spray food over a large area. I had feeble control over keeping my lips closed, so making me laugh when my mouth was full could be disastrous. More food spray. There was the ever-present danger of choking – although there were those who considered that this danger was minimal because of my strong cough reflex.

I had my favourites amongst those who fed me. Imagine my dismay and disgust when there came a diktat from 'on high' that health care assistants were forbidden to feed those with a danger of choking. Trainee nurses were encouraged, however, so a mature, sensible woman, who had come to know and accept my strange habits was replaced by a young, under-confident girl, who perhaps didn't even like what she was doing. I felt more vulnerable – and somewhat exasperated.

Christmas came. My speech therapist had a fund of ideas for making the traditional treats safe. Dried fruits were considered likely to make me choke, but she didn't want me to miss out on the good things. Soaking was her favoured treatment for them. Christmas cake and Christmas pudding could be made soggy with juice, and pudding could be covered with copious amounts of custard or cream. I was allowed soggy food – it was more easily swallowed. I had a better idea for soaking this

Christmas fare – brandy! I felt this was more festive. Punch was quite palatable mixed with thickener, but I wouldn't entertain the possibility of thickening wine.

I was gaining something of a reputation over my relationship with wine. This had been part of our life before the stroke, and I was keen that it should be again. So, when my aunt sent me some money to buy treats for myself, I sent out for some half bottles of wine to have at suppertimes with the exciting mousses (or whatever) sent in by my friend.

It must have seemed quite decadent, alongside the sandwiches and fruit squash enjoyed by the other patients. But it was, I decided, part of my rehabilitation – and in any case I craved one of those sandwiches.

It was, of course, highly disobedient to have a drink without thickener. I also refused thickener in tea and coffee. So at first I only drank fruit juice. Then as time went on some of the nurses consented to let me have tea and coffee, and some of the other rules were relaxed.

I took risks with what I ate right from the start. Risks, that is, in the eyes of the professionals; I never tried anything I didn't think I could cope with. Like a toddler I was continually pushing at the boundaries. I was determined to get back to a normal diet. I would encourage my system in that direction, at my own pace. Boundaries were set regularly by my speech therapist and the 'swallowing expert'. The consistency of food I was allowed, plus the thickness to which my drinks were to be mixed, was specified on a chart and reviewed regularly.

Some of the staff were not happy at all about my flouting the rules, and there ensued a series of discussions over whether I was entitled to make, or indeed capable of making, my own decisions. My speech therapist backed me up on this; she explained the risks of choking and of aspiration pneumonia, then said it was my right to do as I pleased.

Conversely, there was a band of nurses who supported and even applauded my tendency to resist the strictures of authority. It showed a streak of independence and a grim determination that they did not expect in someone so severely affected by stroke.

11. Eating the elephant

Question: 'How do you eat an elephant?'
Answer: 'One bite at a time!'

This was a riddle that we had heard many years before, and which took on a new relevance to what lay before me. The Senior Nursing Officer had said to me: 'you will just have to claw your way back'. The enormity of the task ahead was daunting. I could not afford to look at the big picture – it looked impossible and, quite frankly, terrifying. All I could do was to celebrate each little success and 'keep nibbling away'.

When I started rehabilitation I made myself a timetable of achievements – 'by autumn I shall be transferring; by Christmas I shall be standing; next summer I shall walk out of here', and so on. It did not take very long for me to realise that there was no way I would come anywhere near to achieving those goals. I would have to be thankful for any small improvement and keep 'chewing away at the elephant'! Boy, was it tough and indigestible at times! I was eager to do lots of physical exercises to encourage my useless body to come back to life. But my physiotherapist seemed determined to pursue a 'damage-limitation exercise'. I spent hours having plaster of Paris splints made to fit my legs. When complete, I had to wear them all day every day. Like big, white, rigid, long boots, they were bandaged onto me in the morning and did not come off again till I went to bed at night. I didn't understand the need to prevent deformity at this stage. I got my mother to knit me an oversized pair of socks in garish stripes. I wore them over the splints as a gesture of defiance. My legs and feet were bound and constricted; but my spirit was not . . .

I got extremely frustrated. I wanted to work really hard, to push myself mercilessly. I felt sure that my body would respond.

I became very cross at being told that I was tired and must stop; I wanted to carry on trying. Every day I felt dissatisfied. I thought I was being humoured. I wasn't going to do any good. All that could be done was perhaps to teach me to use a powered wheelchair (which wouldn't be easy). In addition, of course, I had to be helped 'to come to terms' with my new – and limited – future. I did not want to come to terms with anything. This was a temporary situation. It was going to be extremely hard work, but I certainly had no intention of remaining in this condition. Woe betide anyone who suggested otherwise!

I constantly felt that I was 'on trial'. 'Try this', or 'can you do that?' I was challenged. And no, I couldn't. I felt a complete and utter failure. I knew that my situation was dismal. I desperately wanted to feel that the physiotherapist was my ally and together we would fight this demon.

Instead we talked. I use the term 'talked' loosely, because my speech was still vestigial. However my physiotherapist made great efforts to understand my clumsy attempts at communication, and in truth I did find it easier to open my chest and phonate more successfully when lying flat on a physiotherapy couch. So, being a garrulous creature at heart, I did nothing to dissuade – and even encouraged – these conversations, which ranged from news of our respective families to psychological analysis of my situation.

I wanted to exercise hard. I was sure that if I pushed my reluctant body relentlessly hard it was bound to respond. But it didn't seem to work like that. I was given a variety of exercises to do. More often than not I was an abject failure. Nothing seemed to work – actively, that is. Passive movements were easy, even impressive. My years of yoga had stood me in good stead. My joints were very flexible. Someone else could bend them and stretch them to their limits. I could not move them one inch.

It had been decided that it was time for an attempt to be made to teach me to drive the powered wheelchair myself. But I couldn't hold myself upright in one. Neither could I manage any of the standard hand controls designed for the chair which was planned for me. This was established when I was allowed a trial drive. To everyone's horror and alarm, I drove in left-hand circles at high speed, and couldn't slow down, change direction, or turn the motor off.

Clearly this wouldn't do. I was referred to some experts in 'enablement' to see what could be done to improve my chance of driving the wheelchair safely. On the first of several visits to this centre of excellence, I was thoroughly examined by their head physiotherapist to see what, if any, movement I could manage. My joints were flexed and extended to their limits; once again I had cause to be thankful for my years of yoga as my flexibility impressed all who watched.

Unfortunately I was also floppy – I couldn't support my trunk myself, and I was prone to 'spasms'. My muscles would suddenly stretch out (often at the most peculiar angle) and become stiff and immensely strong. Such spasms are a common by-product of severe strokes, often causing great discomfort and pain. Perversely, I actually enjoyed a spasm; I welcomed the sensation of a really good stretch. Later in my rehabilitation I got to know what could initiate these spasms, and took great delight in selectively setting them off, just to feel my muscles tighten up. To prevent these unexpected spasms causing a nasty accident, I would need to be able to switch the chair off instantly. As I couldn't move my hand to the on/off switch, clearly a switch which I could reliably reach and operate was needed. A head switch would fit the bill; my head probably had the best movement of my entire body.

I didn't have the control to drive the chair using the customary spherical knob; I couldn't grip it sufficiently well. So, after some discussion, it was decided that I should try a T-bar instead of the knob on the joystick. I could hold onto that sort of shape with my vice-like grip. Letting go posed a different problem. Relaxing my hand and stretching out my fingers was to provide me with an almost impossible challenge for some years to come. The technician was summoned and given the task of providing me with a removable tray (the right height to support my arms), a head-controlled on/off switch and a T-shaped control bar. Iain was very interested in all this, and enthusiastically discussed all the practicalities and the up-to-date switchery with the technician.

I was told that I was not to drive the wheelchair. The motor had been disconnected from the wheels (a simple matter of flicking a switch) and was supposed to remain so until my physiotherapist deemed that I was 'ready' to be taught. I was indignant. I was not tolerating that. So, not for the only time during my rehabilitation, I took matters into my own hands. The weekend after the wheelchair had been 'customised', Iain and I took to the car park. We had to wait for the weekend because then the physiotherapy department was shut. In the wide open space I practised driving in straight lines and circles, stopping, starting, all in the slowest speed the wheelchair had to offer. I was used to driving a big car (at speed) but this was a different kettle of fish altogether. I had always prided myself on being in complete control; now all I could trust was my head to move side-to-side when I wanted it to, and my right hand to hold the T-bar, fist-like, if someone else moved it into place for me. I could then push from the shoulder, provided that I was braced against the back of the chair, with my head braced against the headrest. But control? By no stretch of the imagination could I claim to be in control of this electric monster! I only had to laugh or cough for one of two things to happen. I tended to go stiff: my legs shot out straight in front of me, my arms became rigid, and either my hand would come off the joystick and I would stop dead, or (more often) I would thrust the joystick forward and crash spectacularly into the wall or whatever happened to be in my way. The idea of the head switch was that I could avoid trouble by switching the machine off quickly whenever a cough or laugh threatened.

One weekend I was practising driving in and out of the spaces between parked cars. Who should come striding across the car park but the director of the rehabilitation unit, my consultant.

"Now I'm for it!" I thought to myself. I had been caught red-handed and expected an admonishment. Gentle and tactful no doubt, but an admonishment all the same. But no! He came over to us both, exchanged a few words with Iain, then praised my progress at manoeuvring the chair. *Aha!* I thought, *If the man at the top gives his blessing, what have I to fear from a physiotherapist's disapproval?* I determined to take more of the initiative in what I did to progress. Caution, I felt, was holding me back.

The nursing staff, on the whole, applauded my efforts to recover. Some were amazed that I had not given up in the face of so many difficulties, and encouraged my independent (belligerent?) attitude. A few, however, failed to hide their displeasure. I should do as I was told, should not make waves, should be 'a good patient'. I was not a good patient! The discomfiture I caused wasn't limited to the occasional nurse. Some of the various therapists found me hard to deal with. There was so much wrong with me: I was paralysed, I couldn't see clearly or speak, and I didn't eat or drink properly. I dribbled, I coughed, and my arms and legs would shoot out stiff and straight without apparent warning. Yet I was mentally sharp, and I had my own ideas about how to effect some sort of recovery. Some people couldn't handle that. I didn't fit into a textbook pattern. Besides, they were the experts, I couldn't possibly know what was best for me, and I shouldn't question their decisions or their behaviour. I, however, considered myself to be the expert on ME, and my nursing background plus many years of doing yoga had given me a basic insight into the workings of the body, and how correct movements of muscles and joints should feel. A few of the 'experts' seemed rather uncomfortable with that. I wasn't an unquestioningly obedient patient. I wanted a say in the rate and manner of my rehabilitation.

I decided that it was time to do something about my appearance. For too long I had allowed myself to be dressed, made up, and my hair done by others, with little or no input from me. Of course this was made worse by my reluctance to look in a mirror. My right eye looked in towards my nose, and I was appalled by my facial appearance. I had never considered myself to be particularly good-looking; now I realised that I should have counted my blessings. I longed to look as I had done before the stroke. I decided to make a list of likes and dislikes for how I wanted to be got ready in the morning. Of course I couldn't do this on my own. I dictated the list to Iain, using a mixture of speech and eye flashes, and he printed it out and stuck it on the wall of my room. This laid me open to all manner of teasing. Some of the nurses already made the effort to comply with my preferences, and could make me comfortable almost by second nature. They regarded my list of 'dos' and 'don'ts' as a huge joke. Those, however, who would have benefited from knowing the way in which I preferred things done, ignored my epistle. Perhaps they were just not interested.

A similar attitude prevailed with regard to communication. My speech therapist was keen to improve communication between me and those who cared for me, while speech was so difficult for me. She arranged several meetings between herself and anyone who worked with me. She and my family had devised a 'formula' for communicating with me. First try proper speech (this was what I wanted to practise). If the listener couldn't make out a word, I should be asked to spell it (again using spoken language), and if that failed I should spell the word using eye flashes (the tried and tested method). This was, I felt, a last resort. Several of the nurses had developed their own, not dissimilar systems. We had formed a good relationship and difficulties were ironed out with good humour. It tended to be these folk who came to the meetings; those who needed some guidance found other pressing tasks to attend to.

It was obvious that I posed all the staff an enormous challenge. My lacking something as fundamental as the ability to speak made the jobs of the nurses, the physiotherapists, the occupational therapists and the psychologists doubly difficult, and for a few it seemed that I had so many problems that I was unlikely to be all there. They treated me accordingly. That made me furious. The speech therapist, I knew, was holding the 'communication meetings' precisely to avoid these unfortunate situations occurring. But I didn't like being the focus of this attention. I was a 'difficult patient'.

I didn't like the thought of being discussed at the nurses' handover meeting. What did I expect? How many hours had I spent in similar meetings when I was nursing, discussing patients' progress? Now I was a patient. Now I was on the receiving end. And I felt very uncomfortable.

Some of the staff remembered that I had a nursing background and chatted to me on relevant topics. Others gave me the impression that I was something of an embarrassment. They would carry out their duties but spend as short a time with me as possible. I confess that I developed a sizeable chip on my shoulder. I wanted to show the world what I had been like before the stroke, so I had some photographs enlarged of me involved in various activities. I had these stuck in a prominent position on my wall. I also wanted people to realise that a lot of that character which they saw in those photographs remained. I became very sensitive about how people spoke to me. I hated feeling patronised. Even unfortunate folk whose way with people was one of naive over attentiveness I regarded as condescending, and I reacted with all the frostiness I could muster.

From a succession of psychologists, there was only one who I thought was on my wavelength; the one who obviously understood how I felt in response to people whom I perceived were patronising me. She did not baulk at discussing the unpleasant and, for some people, unimaginable. We had talked, after all, of the difficulties I would have should I wish to commit suicide. We came to the conclusion that the only way I could take matters into my own hands would be to drive my powered chair along to a busy road and drive headlong into the traffic. Desperate measures! I wasn't that desperate, nor that brave, and have never seriously considered suicide.

My speech therapist considered autonomy and self-advocacy to be very important. She recognised that people with dysphasia (difficulty finding the correct word for a sentence) or dysarthria (difficulty actually forming the words – as I have) tended to be treated as lacking intelligence (which of course they most definitely are not). So several of our sessions were devoted to 'how to get the best out of a situation', 'how to take the initiative in a situation' and 'how to communicate without speech'. I learned a lot: how to position my chair directly in front of the listener for optimum lip reading, how to look alert and in control of the situation, and even how to pre-empt a situation and have a response prepared. The bulk of the time, however, was spent in doing all sorts of repetitive exercises to get my facial muscles, my tongue, my lips and my vocal chords working, and working together. The speech therapist's assistant did these exercises very regularly with me. At one stage she apologised to me because they were repetitive and mundane. She thought I would be bored. Not a bit of it! I enjoyed her company, and besides, I could tell that they were working. True, improvements were neither quick enough nor great enough for my liking, but I had started with nothing so every utterance that sounded vaguely familiar was a bonus.

As my speech became better I learned more techniques for getting a message across, such as rephrasing something which couldn't be deciphered. I also started replacing eye flashes by speech as my favoured method of communication. She, in consultation with members of my family, devised a hierarchy (her term) for people attempting to communicate with me. That, as previously described, consisted of trying normal speech, then spelling out individual words, and failing that, resorting to eye flashes. I was dependent on the listener taking the initiative in changing from one system to another. Otherwise I could continue struggling, unable to make the listener understand. My speech therapist constantly impressed upon me that communication is a two-way process. The onus is just as much on the listener to pay proper attention and to listen carefully, as it is on the speaker to speak clearly and intelligibly. This has been useful advice, despite my tendency to blame myself for being unheard. The nurses closest to me had no need of this 'hierarchy'; they cheerfully made the best of my amateurish mumblings, and we often dissolved in fits of giggles when my attempts at speech were particular gobbledegook. For others, though, my lack of intelligible speech was quite threatening, and having a system of communication in place provided them – and me – with a useful safety-net.

I regarded the physiotherapy sessions as a trial. I always felt under scrutiny. 'Can you do this?' preceded each exercise – and more often than not I couldn't. There was so little I could do. I was given simple movements to practise. I was desperate to succeed; I tried really hard, but my body would not respond. I felt sure that if I put in sufficient effort I could make my muscles work. In fact quite often the harder I tried to move some part of me, the more it refused to co-operate. Nothing I tried to do seemed to do any good, and any movement I did force was discouraged – it was 'the wrong type of movement'. I was incredibly frustrated, and became increasingly bad-tempered. I was disheartened. I considered that my efforts were going unrecognised and unrewarded. I felt let down; I felt abandoned to my fate. I was angry.

The atmosphere between my physiotherapist and me became distinctly frosty. I got on better with other members of the physiotherapy team and – to my shame – made that obvious. There was bad feeling between my other therapists (and nurses) and my physiotherapist: I was often late for other therapy sessions, and all-too-frequently I was left sitting uncomfortably in the wheelchair.

Hydrotherapy was reportedly very beneficial, so I had great expectations of it. Perhaps my expectations were too great, because I was again disappointed in my meagre improvements while in the water. For me the benefits did not outweigh the struggle to get me changed and dried each time.

It was not all failure however. My physiotherapist built a slalom course for me to practise driving my wheelchair with control. I could tell that she was surprised at my proficiency, and that gave me a great deal of satisfaction. My secret driving practice with Iain was paying off! My physiotherapist's aim was to make me capable of coping with a powered wheelchair. This aim had been met. Any further recovery seemed unattainable. I had too many problems. I felt that I had been written off; the task was just too great. No-one had told her how to eat an elephant.

12. Happy birthday

My birthday approached. I was to be allowed home for the day. My only previous excursion had been to the choral society dress rehearsal. Iain had hired a small wheelchair-transporting vehicle, and it had been quite a quick trip out.

None of us had thought that I would ever see home again, so this was quite special. And joy-of-joys, the senior nurse on 'my team' suggested that if this visit were successful, we might aim for weekends at home. It was a very emotional moment when this was put to us. We hadn't dared to hope for this, but it seemed that the situation was already much more optimistic than we had expected. I allowed myself to fantasize about such mundane matters as sitting on our settee, cuddling our cat, and seeing what state the garden was in.

My birthday visit went pretty well. We had friends and family to a small party in the garden, and I was able to explore all the downstairs rooms in the house. I revelled in the familiar sights and smells; parts of my life I had feared were lost to me.

But it was at home that I suffered an enormous emotional setback. I had set my heart on sitting on the settee. I fully expected that with the help of a person on either side of me I would be able to step out of the wheelchair, turn, and sit down on the settee. The family were very dubious. I was adamant. So we tried. It didn't feel right as I tried to stand. My legs would not take my weight. I crumpled. If Iain and both daughters had not held on to me I would have fallen. They lifted me bodily – and not without difficulty – onto the settee. I was somewhat chastened. I was very disappointed. Recovery was not going to be merely a matter of determination. My body would no longer obey my brain. I was no longer master of my actions.

On my return to the rehabilitation centre I was subdued and depressed. This was going to be an enormous, perhaps impossible task to achieve. For a while I forgot about 'little bites'.

This elephant was far too big to tackle!

However, that day at home was fortunately just the start. Iain and I had to have a rehearsal in the flat belonging to the rehabilitation centre. There we could spend the night and day ostensibly on our own, yet with help nearby should we need it. We had to ensure that we could manage all the equipment and other trappings of life with a paralysed person. Of course it was Iain who bore the brunt of the physical effort and the responsibility involved. We passed the test, and so the stage was set for me to spend weekends at home. Before this could become a reality, however, there were some changes to be made to the house. For a start, I needed a bedroom downstairs. Our bedroom and the dining room had to be swapped. Table, chairs, and best china all went upstairs. Down came our bed and the contents of the bathroom cupboard. Then a ramp had to be built so that I could get in and out of the house. Lastly, the social service department had to be requested to supply various items of equipment – a hoist, bedpan, and portable ramps, and to provide professional carers when required.

Then there was the matter of transport. In the short term we could hire the small wheelchair-carrying vehicle – but that was fairly costly, and in any case we couldn't go anywhere as a family in it; it was too small. We needed a vehicle of our own. Our beloved Volvo estate would have to go. I had enjoyed driving that car. I had enjoyed driving per se. But now I was unfit to drive and was legally obliged to surrender my licence. That was hard. I had been driving since my seventeenth birthday, and it was an important part of my life. I felt that by sending my licence back I was admitting that I would never drive again, and that part of my life had disappeared – or possibly had not even existed.

I was having difficulty equating the 'pre-stroke me' with the 'me now'. It was as if the person I once was had disappeared – maybe, I was afraid, disappeared without trace. The photographs of myself I had up on the wall were of the things I most enjoyed: playing the piano, cooking, standing on my head. Perhaps more for my own benefit than for others', it was a reminder that this was the same person, and everything I had done or been before remained an important part of who I was now. I didn't try to discuss this with the psychologists as I considered my feelings on the matter to be too complicated. Silly really: that's what the psychologists were there for.

Weekends at home were something more than we had dared hope for. They gave me a degree of freedom, and I felt I was a 'proper' member of the family again. In addition, I could try out things I 'wasn't allowed' – to eat or to do – in the rehabilitation centre. I had been craving chips for as long as I could remember – well before I could eat at all – but they were deemed too difficult for me to chew and swallow. So one day when I was at home, we had fish and chips for supper. What a treat! It took a large amount of tomato ketchup to make them moist enough to manage, but I had fantasized long enough; I was determined not to miss out.

A while later, I sat on a proper toilet for the first time. At home. I was held up by being attached to the hoist. That would not have been allowed in the rehabilitation centre; officially it was misuse of the equipment. I was not averse to breaking rules if I thought they were hampering my progress.

Iain did some research and visited a few specialist vehicle sellers, and soon we were the owners of a van big enough to transport me, three passengers and a generous amount of luggage. It had been adapted to take me in the wheelchair, and I got into it via the side door by driving up a ramp which spent most of the time slung underneath. Initially I was pushed up the ramp and into position, but as I became more confident at driving the chair, I took myself up the ramp and manoeuvred into place, before the chair was anchored down to the floor of the van, and I was strapped in, for complete safety. Not for the fainthearted to watch – I presented quite a spectacle, driving up an incline not much wider than the wheelbase of the chair, and turning around in an extremely confined space, nearly two feet from the ground. Even more hair-raising than entering the van was getting out of it, as I had to come out backwards. I had to put my trust in whomever was helping to navigate me out safely.

Although I resented 'the van' (as it quickly became known), because I felt it was a badge of my disability, it gave us as a family independence and mobility, and allowed us to start opening up my life (and our lives) once more. I began going home most weekends. We visited friends, and had outings to local places of interest, to concerts and so on. More importantly perhaps, when our elder daughter started university over a hundred miles away I was able to accompany the rest of the family to take her and see her settled in.

One evening when Iain was staying with me, he read to me some of his feelings, jotted down during the early days following the stroke. It was fascinating to hear another perspective on events. I began to recall all my changing emotions at such an upheaval – such a rude interruption to all of our lives. I determined to write a book about my experiences. There had been a dearth of literature to give me encouragement. In the early days Iain had trawled the internet for any relevant technical information. This was very dry, full of statistics, and in some cases frankly depressing. I had felt very alone. I would write a book so that no-one else need feel alone, however dark the circumstances.

Except that I couldn't write. Someone would have to write for me. The occupational therapy department possessed an aged computer and 'my' occupational therapist offered to type my prose into the word processor. So I 'dictated' to her: first using eye flashes then, when I began to speak more, using words. It was extremely time-consuming. The computer was old and slow, and although dictating was good speech therapy practice, this was an unsatisfactory way to proceed. Iain decided that my Christmas present would be a computer of my own. There was a telephone socket in my room, so I would be able to use e-mail to get back in touch with the world. The staff agreed to my having my own phone-line, and were very enthusiastic about my literary plans. There was just one drawback to this plan: I couldn't use a keyboard. Or a mouse. The only part of my two hands and arms that I could use was my right thumb, and that had limited movement. How could I hope to use a computer?

Once again, Iain came up trumps. He researched the problem and found a computer program which ran an on-screen keyboard. This could be operated by a switch, strapped to my hand and controlled by that right thumb. I had to ask to be connected up, and for the computer to be switched on. Once that was done I could enter a different world. A world in which I was articulate, where no-one knew that I was paralysed, where I could be my old self – on paper at least. Iain spent many hours setting it all up for me to use. He made as much as possible happen automatically at the click of the switch. At last I had cause to be grateful for his almost fanatical interest in all things electronic. Everything seemed incredibly complex, yet he sat patiently working, making it possible to operate the computer with the use of one thumb and a small electronic switch. I quickly mastered the techniques of scanning the 'keyboard' for the letter I required then clicking the switch to 'type', and of moving the cursor around by means of a set of little arrows at the corner of the screen.

My day took on some purpose. When there was no therapy scheduled, instead of watching television (the other main option) I would write 'my book', or write letters – and later when the phone line was connected, e-mails. Life (after a fashion) began again. I could 'speak' to the world, I had a task to complete, and best of all, I had a modicum of independence – something I had not known since that dreadful day in March. For many years I had despised computers; I had scorned people's dependence on them, and resented the amount of time 'wasted' on their use. Now I had cause to be extremely thankful for their existence.

Around this time I learned another 'skill': that of silk painting. Or rather silk splodging, for that is what it was. The leisure activities were 'under new management'. The occupational therapist who tried to make me into a mouth painter had moved on and had been replaced by a much more down-to-earth and sensible person, so I felt less inclined to play truant (as I had been wont to do). I was assigned to work with the OT assistant, and over the months we built up an easy-going and productive relationship. She very quickly caught on that I wanted to get some use of my right hand, and suggested activities that would give it some exercise. Among other things, I painted several multi-coloured silk scarves as presents for proud relatives, and towards the end of my stay in the rehabilitation centre I was asked to paint some (very impressionistic) silk pictures, which were exhibited and subsequently sold. Fame at last! I also went shopping with this lady – my first 'independent' (if they can be called that) forays into the city. I was terribly self-conscious – about my appearance, about my inability to speak properly;

setting aside the fact of my paralysis and all that entailed for negotiating pavements, roadways and shops. But I had to 'bite the bullet' – being a recluse for the rest of my life was not an option. Being out with me did not seem to cause my escort any embarrassment (I felt sure that it must) and for this I felt very grateful, and not a little humble.

I was equally thankful for the equanimity of my family. None of them seemed uncomfortable at being 'seen out' with me whether at the supermarket or a concert.

13. With a little help from my friends

This chapter runs the risk of becoming like a theatrical awards ceremony: 'I would like to thank . . .' (and a long list of names)! I will attempt to avoid that. But it is my firm conviction that a strong support network is vital to tackle a crisis of this magnitude. It is not something which one can face alone.

I consider myself very fortunate in that not only was my support network immensely strong; it is close-knit. I was not (and am not) short of support and well-wishers. Some of the latter came from very surprising quarters and with astonishing intensity and generosity.

For the first few days following the stroke, when it was doubtful that I would survive, Iain received a number of letters of condolence such as one might expect on the death of a partner. As time went on, however, and I did not die, he started receiving letters expressing sympathy for the plight in which we now found ourselves. Very soon I was inundated with cards and notes sending me optimistic messages. I have already described the huge numbers of flowers arriving for me while I was in ITU which had to go straight home. They continued to arrive as I moved on and could keep them with me. I was not without flowers at any time up until the day I went home. Presents too; I received audiotapes of poetry, short stories and music. People gave me books of inspiring biographies. Others pampered me with luxuries. Two, however, made a lasting impression upon me. The first was a letter from an old friend. In it she expressed her feeling of helplessness, and that the most meaningful thing she felt she could do was to go into her church and say a special Mass on my behalf. The other was from a couple who had taught our daughters. They sent me their most treasured possession – a set of audiotapes recounting the life of a man of great importance within their faith. They wanted me to accept this as a gift. I was overwhelmed by their generosity and selflessness. But I could not keep their precious possession. I listened to the tapes, then returned them with a letter of explanation and gratitude. I felt humbled by the messages of support; not only from those close to me but also people who knew of me only by name. Humbled and strengthened! Various people down the years have doubted that I could keep my faith when such a catastrophe happened in church of all places, and on Mothering Sunday of all days.

My faith was undoubtedly altered, but it was certainly still kept. I could see God at work in so many ways, through so many people.

I learnt the true meaning of faithfulness during those first few months. Not a day went past, barely a waking minute, without Iain there at my side. Whenever an unpleasant procedure was planned, he would be there to hold my hand. I trusted him implicitly, and knew that I could depend on him to 'fight my corner'. Even when I was an inert, unresponsive lump, he would greet me and say goodbye with a kiss; and he always talked to me normally (and encouraged others to do likewise), as if I was totally aware of what was going on. Which, of course, I was. What steadfast and loyal belief he showed in me. I was glad to prove that belief justified – at least in part.

Our daughters, too, were steadfast in their loyal support. In the early days I would spend my first waking moments expectantly watching the door into the ITU. I didn't have to wait long. Without fail, Iain would appear, accompanied either by one of our daughters or by my mother – she likewise diligently kept a vigil (we were allowed just two visitors at a time, so my family took turns to be at my side). After I had been transferred to the main ward they arranged their visits in shifts, so that one of them was always with me. This gave me great confidence. I was dependent on Iain and our girls to be my advocates, and I felt very vulnerable without them. They would 'listen' to me. I could rely on that.

Our wider family and our friends were also very supportive. Some of my friends were around at the start, and offered comfort to my family as well as to me. Both family and friends provided practical help and support to Iain and to our girls, for example giving them a good meal on a regular basis. In retrospect I feel I was rather ungracious – and I was certainly vain – when some of my friends asked if they might visit me. I said 'No'. I didn't want them to see me in such a state, and firmly believed that this was a temporary predicament and I would soon look my old self again. They may have been hurt; they may have been secretly relieved – I have no inkling – but to their credit they stood by me and waited until I felt ready to see them. Other friends had no such compunction (for which I remain humbled and grateful) and were there at the start – and remained so thereafter. Yet others whom I had not seen for many years either came to see me or got in touch, so I was not short of support or good wishes.

But what of the professionals? Like all people, I found some personalities were more appealing than others. I also judged their professional skills. I couldn't help it; old habits die hard, and I wasn't as insensible as some considered me.

I don't have many memories of the staff in ITU and the High Dependency Unit – presumably because I was there a relatively short time, and during much of that time my head was full of hallucinations. But I remember being impressed that the nursing staff always spoke to me before doing anything to me. They introduced themselves, explained what they were about to do, and generally exuded an air of calm. One who stood out from all the rest was a Canadian nurse (she had a distinctive accent) whose manner was so soothing and capable that she inspired in me a feeling of confidence and security. The fact that she shared a – very unusual – name with my grandmother made her doubly special.

The medical staff, however, were a different matter. On the whole, that is, for there are of course exceptions. Doctors would discuss me and my condition within my earshot, and these discussions seemed to be very negative in their nature. This made me very angry. Did they think I couldn't hear? Or didn't understand? Or was it just that they didn't think? I couldn't respond, nor could I react. I felt that I was being 'written off'. But not only that. The professional in me was furious at their behaviour. They must surely have known that it was extremely bad practice to discuss a patient within earshot, whatever his or her apparent state of consciousness. I was not impressed (but having said that, it was probably useful to hear what they really thought; it just served to strengthen my resolve to fight).

I moved to the ward via the High Dependency Unit (after a false start when I was moved with my condition still unstable, and had to be returned as an emergency for closer care). There, there seemed to have been so many changes since the days when I worked on the wards. For a start, there was no ward sister. Instead, the nursing staff workforce was divided into 'teams', each with a 'team leader'. There appeared to be no-one in overall charge. This was anathema to me. There was no obvious hierarchy either. Newly-qualified nurses were indistinguishable (initially at least) from those with years of experience – and corresponding competence and confidence. Old-fashioned to the core, I found this very unsettling. I didn't approve. But what did that matter any more? My nursing days were over. I was 'a patient'.

Of course there were some nurses of whom I became very fond. Some personalities whom I took to more readily. Some whose skills and conscientiousness were impressive and humbling. Some on whose presence I began to depend. Several of the qualified nurses fell into that category, and there was a health care assistant who was very important to me. She left to do nursing training. She was an excellent candidate, and would do well, I felt. I applauded her decision.

There was one nurse who neatly provided an illustration of one of the major problems following a stroke: that of inappropriate behaviour. Something about his demeanour must have amused me when I first saw him, because every time he had cause to approach me or even speak to me, I would burst into fits of uncontrollable laughter. It was funny at first, but it soon became an embarrassment – and it must have been very wearing for him. But I couldn't stop myself (I couldn't talk, but I could laugh – and loudly, at that). Apart from the occasional sarcastic comment, he bore it very well.

The nurses from other nations were a mixed blessing. Their value was largely dependent upon their grasp of English and English habits. That influenced their understanding of not only their patients, but also the instructions given about their care. Imagine my horror when one nurse began to force my medication into the wrong part of my gastrostomy tube. A sizeable amount of liquid, she should have put it down the main bore of the tube, straight into my stomach. I was powerless to stop her putting it down the part of the tube used for filling the small balloon that held the tube in place. As she forced this large amount of liquid into the small (and already full!) balloon, she ignored the shaking of my head and my frantic eye-movements, until a sharp 'POP' suggested to her that something was wrong. Too late! I was furious. With the balloon burst, there was nothing to keep the tube in place. There was no time to waste. Before the tube fell out, and the opening started to heal over, it had to be replaced and secured. This was a tricky procedure, and unpleasant for me. I was unimpressed that it was made necessary.

Of the rest of the hospital staff, I think with fondness of the two physiotherapists who visited me every day. The junior of the two came every morning to 'stretch' my limbs. This involved a series of passive exercises to keep my muscles stretched and my joints flexible. Her fear was that the exercises might cause me pain. But in truth I enjoyed them. I welcomed the sensations of moving the joints and stretching the muscles; it was actually quite soothing. One of the nurses on the night shift made a point of fitting this exercise routine into her care schedule if I was awake, and I was very grateful for that.

Later, the two physiotherapists paid me a daily visit with the tilt table for a further exercise session. An army of ward staff slid me across onto it and I was strapped into place. Getting vertical was a gradual process. For several days I was only taken to a slight angle, then as time progressed and I became more 'acclimatised' I was taken to a more perpendicular position. Here I was given various exercises to carry out, such as turning my head from side to side and tilting each ear towards the corresponding shoulder,

All too soon, so it seemed, it was decided that I should sit out of bed. I didn't want to leave the security of my bed. I was introduced to the indignities of the hoist. I felt like a freight package as I swung from my bed to the adjacent chair. It felt very odd (in particular my head felt very dizzy) to be seated in a chair after several weeks of lying, and then being propped up, in bed. Then it was time to progress to the wheelchair, in which I was taken out and about. The physiotherapists were intent that I should get 'moving' again as quickly as possible. I was not to languish any more than was necessary. However, although they were hard taskmasters, I became quite fond of them. They dealt kindly with my tantrums (oh yes, I did have those), gave me lots of helpful hints and praised even the smallest of my achievements or improvements, and for me that assumed a surprising degree of importance.

I received an amazing number of visitors while I was in the hospital. Friends whom I had not seen for years arrived. Names from Christmas cards and birthday cards and an annual letter acquired faces once more as their owners appeared at my bedside. I had regular visits from a number of my faithful friends and relations. That, together with the daily presence of Iain and one or both daughters, meant that I never felt neglected. I continued to be visited regularly after my move to the rehabilitation centre. My family became quite familiar to the nursing staff, and over the twelve months that I was there they developed an easy-going, even close, relationship with some of them.

Of course I had my favourites. I formed quite close friendships with a handful of the nurses. They seemed to understand my feeble attempts at speaking. They saw beyond my multiple shortcomings and treated me as a fellow professional; this went a long way to making me feel better about myself. I could not bear to see myself in a mirror because of my stiff and distorted face, with the right eye pointing towards my nose. My coughing, snorting, grunting and dribbling also caused me great anguish. That was apart from my complete paralysis and inability to converse properly. I felt that these ladies were the only ones who could sit me comfortably in my wheelchair, or feed me 'correctly'. Whenever one of them was on duty I felt confident and safe. If none were around, I felt exceedingly vulnerable.

Vulnerable is how I felt at my physiotherapy sessions. As I've said previously, I desperately wanted to try hard to make things work, but either my body wouldn't co-operate or 'my' physiotherapist wouldn't allow me to because I would encourage 'the wrong type of movement'. I felt a complete failure, and all my problems appeared to be such a disappointment. It seemed that expectations for any recovery were very low and 'damage limitation' was the aim of my treatment. I was always relieved when some of the others (and one in particular) treated me, and my making it so obvious was disloyal. I was admonished. 'My' physiotherapist did her best to be 'chummy' with me, to build a relationship with me. It was just a misfitting of personalities. I was glad to return to my friends, the nurses, or to go to my next 'class' – which was usually speech therapy. I counted my speech therapist and her assistant among my 'favourites'. The assistant, in particular, was immensely patient with me. It was an uphill struggle to enable me to talk again. The three main areas involved in speech (i.e. the muscles of face and mouth, the throat and vocal chords, the lungs and respiratory tract) all needed considerable work. There was nothing for it but to do the same repetitive exercises day after day; these she did with me with untold patience and good humour. I have cause to be extremely grateful to these two ladies – not only because they taught me that effective communication is not solely a matter of clear speech.

One more member of staff brightened up my days. After the initial debacle at the 'leisure' group in occupational therapy, where they tried to make me paint with my head, one of the assistants got the message that I wanted to exercise my right hand. In addition, a couple of games of Scrabble made it obvious that I was still in possession of my faculties. After that we got on famously, and had a few projects together. It was she who made the silk painting a success, and it was she who took me shopping in the city. She showed me that it could be done – albeit with some forward planning. I could go shopping. It was a slower and more complicated exercise than it had been before, but the hassles involved were far outweighed by the pleasure I derived from going into a shop and personally choosing something. She even took me for a drink in a café; something I had thought I would never do again.

But it was being able to use my computer that gave me the most independence. In print I was lucid and intelligible and my old friends could have a mental picture of the old me. How different from the inarticulate and inert creature whom they encountered when they visited.

14. The home run

We were due to leave the RAF in less than a year when I had my stroke. So, soon Iain would be jobless, and we would be homeless. After the initial crisis had passed, it was imperative to give this some attention. The plan was that Iain should work in medical education, with a part-time post as a GP.

When he had jobs lined up, then we could start the hunt for a home. For so many years I had dreamt of house hunting. Of looking for the ideal place for the rest of our lives, and making it our own. Instead I would have to delegate that adventure (responsibility?) to Iain and one of our daughters. But first 'we' needed a job!

We were both very disappointed when, about 7 months after the stroke, Iain failed to secure an education job in the nearest city, but soon after he was offered one in the East of England, a part of the country with which we were not familiar. This was indeed going to be an adventure. One in which I was to be a passive player. Our next task was to scour the medical press every week, on the lookout for an advertisement for a suitable job in general practice. We didn't have to wait long. Nor could we believe our luck. There, staring us in the face, was an advertisement for a half-time GP. All the criteria we wished for in a future job for Iain were fulfilled. This was meant to be, it seemed.

Iain applied for the partnership, and he got it. He was highly delighted. From despondency to delight in such a short time . . .

We now had to turn our attention to finding somewhere to live. We had certain requirements which would narrow our choice of properties quite considerably. No longer could we consider an old property needing improvement, perhaps on several floors, and with a large garden. Not only had we to consider ease of access, but there was the not inconsiderable fact that I would be unable to contribute to our new home either financially or physically. It was up to Iain and Elisabeth (on her school holiday) to comb the local estate agents and make a shortlist of suitable places for me to peruse. Meanwhile, I continued with my rehabilitation. I felt that I was making some headway with my speech exercises. Steady progress, yet very slow. On the physiotherapy front, however, I could see little improvement. I felt very frustrated as I considered that I should be worked harder. I had my suspicions that it had been decided that I had reached the limit of my recovery. I felt sure that I hadn't. As if to reinforce this, I surprised my physiotherapist by demonstrating better-than-adequate control of my powered wheelchair. That gave me great satisfaction. The nursing staff were, as ever, supportive and encouraging. Those I counted as friends followed our house hunting with great interest and involvement. Iain and Elisabeth reported back to me with arms full of property details, most of which were totally unsuitable. A handful, however, were worth a look, so a 'day out' was planned. An early start was necessary, as we had a long way to go. The night staff dressed me for my outing. They had quite a struggle with some of my clothes; it became rapidly apparent that fitted clothes were impossible now and that I was going have to wear stretch or elasticated fabrics. It was a lack-lustre selection of houses that was lined up for me to inspect. Each one would have needed alterations made to fit our changed circumstances, and they all required smartening-up, but eventually we decided on one. It seemed to be sufficiently spacious and would need the minimum alteration for me to cope with it.

I returned to the rehabilitation centre, we made an offer (which was accepted), and we awaited the results of the building survey.

We received them a short while later. We were horrified to discover that the house had got some major structural problems; so major that we considered the house to be potentially dangerous. We dropped it like a hot potato – much to the chagrin of the vendor. So there we were, back at square one again.

Meanwhile, I could feel myself becoming more and more

institutionalised. While my family worried about becoming homeless, I was quite content cocooned as I was from the outside world. I watched people re-learn to use the telephone, to use buses and trains, to cope in shops; all beyond me. I was going to need assistance with absolutely everything – and that dependence was fast becoming a habit. I waited to be given a drink, to have the switch for my computer attached to my hand, to have my mail read to me. I was waited upon on a scale that would previously have been totally unacceptable, unthinkable, and I was becoming comfortable with it. It had to stop. Quite how, I had not yet fathomed out. Perhaps a few more rules had to be broken. I had to stop being complacent and push a few more boundaries.

A new shortlist of possible homes was being prepared. At the same time, Iain compiled video footage for me of the market town that was to be his workplace and possibly our home. All roads in and out were featured, together with the town centre shops and the surgery. I was still having problems with my eyesight, so it was hard to appreciate, but it did help a bit.

Around this time (and not for the first time) it was put to me that I should have a **suprapubic catheter** inserted instead of the **urethral** one I had had in place from the start. For this, a small hole is made in the lower abdomen, just above the pubic bone and the catheter is passed directly into the bladder. This has the advantage of leaving the perineum unencumbered. I had so far resisted this, as in my previous experience as a nurse, a suprapubic catheter was a permanent feature, and I categorically rejected that idea. I listened with some cynicism to the nurses' protestations of its non-permanence, but I had to secretly admit that it was going to be a great deal more difficult to get rid of this tube than it had been disposing of the tracheostomy and the gastrostomy tubes. So I agreed to join the waiting list for this surgical procedure; at the same time the surgeons would remove a sizeable bladder stone which was causing problems.

In the event, I found the new catheter more comfortable than the urethral one. I got used to having a hole in my abdomen and a small dressing surrounded the catheter and covered the hole. I could now sit more comfortably and my clothing didn't pull it. Pride prevented me from admitting that it would have been sensible to have had the catheter moved sooner.

More surgery was in the offing. Regular visits to the ophthalmologist had culminated in him offering to operate on my right eye. If we were very fortunate, straightening the eye (by shortening its lateral muscle) would 'lock' its image into that of the left. Thus the double vision would be eliminated. Even if that didn't work totally, the cosmetic effect would be worth it. I hated the way I looked. But once again I had to wait.

It was time to make another trip to look at houses. Another early start: we were heading for a village a few miles from the surgery. There were several houses on our list, one of which was still under construction. I had studied the plans of it, and it looked quite promising.

We saved that one until last, and found the first on our list much as the others had been: uninspiring, but possible – if we were prepared to make some structural alterations. We were beginning to lose heart, and 'wandered' along the road to examine the building site. And building site it certainly was; with its high metal fence, and piles of bricks amongst the mud. But I had a good feeling about it. Iain thought it looked small, but I remembered the measurements written on the plans and if they were accurate then the place would be far from small. It was true that the garden would be smaller than we had originally (in normal circumstances) planned, but I was now unable to do my share of gardening, so that was not such a bad thing. I felt – rightly or wrongly – that the onus was on me for a decision. So I made one. The building site was for us. So I was taken back to the rehabilitation centre, and all the administrative arrangements fell to Iain.

Now we had somewhere to live – or rather, would have once the house was finished. Meanwhile, my rehabilitation had to continue. I was working hard at speech therapy, and constantly worried the nurses and speech therapists alike because I insisted on eating and drinking 'unsuitable' foods. My swallowing was still deemed inadequate for such things as baked potatoes and toast. I refused to have thickener in tea or coffee – or wine. I still was not happy with physiotherapy and hydrotherapy (apparently everyone's panacea) was particularly disappointing. In occupational therapy I continued to turn out silk paintings: their abstract nature made them quite successful. My passion for cooking had to be diverted to teaching my younger daughter. She did not need much teaching, but communication with her was a useful speech therapy exercise.

I began to replace my eye flashes with 'proper' speech as my main method of communication. This was not without its problems. For all that I was working on my articulation, the volume of my speech was almost non-existent. Anything I did manage to say was in a flat monotone. Calling out and shouting were out of the question. In my head the words sounded perfectly clear, but it was not so for the listeners. It was quite a challenge, and one had to pay close attention to my conversation to decipher what I was saying. What did make my blood boil was people pretending that they had understood what I had said when they patently had not. The glazed expression, plus the mumbled 'uh-huh' or 'Mmmm' were something of a giveaway. I much preferred it if people said 'look, I didn't understand a word of that'. Perhaps they were being kind . . .

Another thing that made me angry was that when some people did not understand what I said they would either ignore me (seemingly considering my utterances to be of little import) or cast their eyes around the room, trying to guess what I might have said. Many a time I have known the answer to the question 'where is . . .?', but after several unsuccessful attempts at communicating that knowledge I have mentally shrugged and thought: *What the hell*, and left the enquirer to his or her own devices. Perhaps the question was a rhetorical one. It was certainly treated as if it were . . .

There were yet more days out for choosing such things as kitchen units and wall and floor tiles. It would have been so exciting under different circumstances, but knowing that it would be someone other than me using the kitchen and taking care of the house somewhat took the edge off my enthusiasm. The house was coming on, and Iain had started his new jobs. He was living in a little bungalow belonging to the doctor whom he was replacing. While I was regularly assured that I would not be made homeless from the rehabilitation centre, it was time to consider a move to the area of the country which was going to become home. Behind the scenes there were frantic negotiations to that end, but I was ignorant of these at the time.

One day, seemingly out of the blue, I was given the news

that I would be leaving the rehabilitation centre. This came as quite a shock – and not just to me. My speech therapist and her assistant still had plans for work that we should do. They clearly didn't think that their job was done. And I was just about to enter some of my silk paintings (under the auspices of the occupational therapy assistant, who had become such an encouragement to me) in an exhibition of hospital patients' artwork. The physiotherapist, however, evidently considered that I had reached 'the end of the road'. I was very upset. I had wanted (unreasonably and unrealistically) to leave rehabilitation in the same condition as I had been eighteen months previously, before the stroke. I knew all about strokes and their consequences. But I was different, wasn't I? I had survived and come this far, hadn't I? Why no further? It took a great deal of soul-searching and discussion (or the nearest approximation I could manage) to come to terms with leaving in this 'condition'. This did not have to be 'it'. I could continue to improve in the months – and even years – ahead.

I was to be moved to a small hospital closer (though not close) to our new home. It was a rehabilitation unit for the elderly, with one of its wards devoted to respite care. I was put on this ward until our house was ready (or so I was told).

My arrival must have shocked the staff of this respite ward. I had with me my computer (for which I requested a telephone connection so that I could use email), several pieces of furniture and all manner of 'bits and pieces'. The wherewithal for a veritable home from home, as I had had in the rehabilitation centre. This was obviously not what was expected of a patient. Neither were my attempts at independence. I was admonished for straying too far from the ward when I set off to explore the attractive grounds. It very quickly became apparent that the ethos of this 'respite' unit was very different from that of the 'rehabilitation' unit I had left. Some of the staff applauded my independence of spirit, and encouraged me to continue. Others, however, were clearly uncomfortable with my demeanour and tried to make me conform to the model of a 'good' patient. Unsuccessfully. Whether cleaners, health care assistants, qualified nurses, or medical staff: there were those who saw beyond my paralysis and poor speech to the intelligent, spirited woman who wanted to defy as many of the stroke's constraints as possible.

Then there were those who became most upset if I wanted to take risks, who wanted me just to do as I was told and 'not rock the boat'. Again I felt that to some I was a lost cause. It was the occupational therapist who seemed to have the best understanding of my situation: suggesting that I must feel imprisoned in my useless body. That was just how it felt. Although it was almost automatic to rail against it, the only constructive way I could see of dealing with it was to try to build a life within the many constraints placed upon me.

All this time, the builders were busy. The house was almost finished. There were choices to be made, finishing touches to be decided upon. There could be no more weekends at home. I could have days out to the new house or to the tiny bungalow in which was Iain was living. I felt that I was 'treading water', making no progress. Waiting for our new home to be ready.

I was not short of visitors. My friends continued to come – and I could even hold some sort of conversation with them. The same applied to members of my family. Some were better than others at interpreting my feeble attempts at speech. For feeble they were! Of the three components of speech (articulation, phonation and breath support), although none were adequately proficient, my worst was at breath support. I just did not have any 'puff'.

Consequently my voice (such as it was) was practically inaudible. A gadget called a 'speech amplifier' was deemed necessary, and the speech therapist busied herself finding a suitable one for me. In the event, one was specially made for me. It consisted of a small microphone which was to be worn on a thin metal collar around my neck. The batteries and the loudspeaker were housed in a box, not unlike a cigarette packet in size and shape. This was designed to go in a pocket. It was not a success for two main reasons. Firstly, not only speech was amplified. All upper-body noises became magnified. And I wasn't short of those. Burps, slurps, grunts and sighs. They were all made obvious, and couldn't be ignored or disguised. Secondly, imperfect speech was amplified just as readily as perfect articulation, so I was no more intelligible. I did not like it. Not for the first time, I vowed to manage without gadgets.

It meant hard work for me, and possibly harder work for my listeners, but I felt that was preferable to reliance on an electronic device.

A succession of professional people providing support at home came to see me. A social worker came to discuss my care during the day and overnight. An assessment of the number of hours of social care I required (for that is what it is called) was made, negotiated between Iain, me and the social worker because I was deemed to be in need of 24-hour care. The county in which we were about to live was pioneering a scheme whereby, instead of receiving the prescribed care from social service staff, the 'client' would receive sufficient funds to employ his or her own staff. This meant that I could employ whomever I wanted, to work the hours I chose. Furthermore, there was a team who would administer all this if I so wished. I had a visit from a member of this team to explain how it all worked.

Yet another visitor came to organise the 'environmental controls' that I would have at home. How I hated that term. It was completely irrational but I am sure that my dislike of the name contributed to my initial resistance. I preferred to think of them as 'remote controls', not unlike that of the TV.

Up until then I had been using a fixed switch on a large machine which operated an alarm, a light and the TV volume and channel. I decided that I would do better with the small, portable box. This new system was the deluxe model, with three times as many functions. I could use it while mobile in my chair and would be able to operate the TV, radio and stereo, an intercom, the telephone, various lights and several electric sockets of my choice. There was even the promise of an electronic door-opener. Such independence!

Yet another visitor was an official from social services, to see which items of equipment I would need at home and to arrange for their supply. In addition the head of the Community Rehabilitation Team paid me a visit. It was her job to enumerate the services that the team would be offering me on my discharge home. Everything seemed to be getting organised for me to go home. I was even to have my own tilt table. This seemed daring; so far I had only been allowed on the tilt table under the supervision of the physiotherapists. The physiotherapists and I had

had a difficult relationship. I always wanted to do more work, to take more risks. They concentrated on playing things safe. I could never be sure for whose benefit this was – mine or theirs. But now I was to have a tilt table of my own. One was ordered for me. I was allowed to choose the colour.

Very soon, it seemed, the house was finished and we took it over from the builder amid much celebration (I was allowed a day out for the occasion).

One of my fellow patients gave me good advice on where best to go for soft furnishings, so on another day out we went and chose carpets and curtains and arranged for their fitting.

It was all coming together. Now we only needed to decide on and arrange a moving date. With alarm, I noted that the subject of my discharge seemed to have been shelved. I was given various lame excuses as to why a decision on my discharge date could not be made. I was enraged! After over twenty years of marriage we were about to have our own home and I didn't intend missing out on moving in. Of course, it would be very different from how over the years we had envisaged settling down in our own home. I wouldn't be moving furniture into place, or unpacking boxes. I would have to be content with supervising (that term was frequently cropping up now) and deciding what was to go where. However, it was a much better situation than might have been. At one stage it was feared that I might never come home. Then the hope became that I could come home but be tube-fed and unable to speak at all. So this was more than we had hoped for. But whenever I enquired about my possible discharge I received noncommittal replies: 'you will need such-and-such in place' and 'this or that isn't ready' were typical responses. This just wasn't good enough. I wanted to be – intended that I should be – involved in the move as far as was practically possible. What was I to do?

I remembered some advice given by my speech therapist at the rehabilitation centre. People with dysarthria could pre-empt discussion and difficult questioning by writing a list of the points they would make should they be able to speak effectively.

So I set to on my word-processor and compiled a page full of reasons why I should be discharged. There were some practicalities which I had to cover. I asked our daughters if they would provide the personal care I needed until social services could get their care package in place. They readily agreed. I felt very humbled. Caring for me would involve doing things which I would never have expected anyone to do for me, let alone my children. But they weren't children anymore. And now the tables were turned. It was I who had to be cared for. *How the mighty have fallen* kept running through my mind. I asked for a meeting with the powers-that-be about my immediate future. I wasn't going to be stalled any longer . . .

The day of the meeting dawned. I had ensured that my whole family could be with me. I also ensured that I had lots of copies of my 'statement of intent' as I privately called it. Those present included representatives from social services, the Community Rehabilitation Team, occupational therapy and physiotherapy – as well as nursing staff. They were all given a copy. Any objections any of them might have had, or complications they might have raised, were dealt with by what I had written. I had taken the wind out of everyone's sails. What I had feared would be a long drawn out affair was in fact a businesslike matter of deciding who needed to organise what in order for me to be discharged on the date I had suggested. I would need a hoist and a shower chair immediately, but the environmental controls could wait. My daughters would need some assistance from social service carers at first, but I could start the process of employing my own staff as soon as I got home. We already had a suitable vehicle and Iain (with help where necessary from the social worker) organised all the financial benefits to which I was entitled.

I was excited. I would be going home. After almost a year and a half in institutions. And it was to be to our own home – for the first time in 23 years of married life.

There was the small matter of a moving-in date. After some strong discussion with the family, we reached the compromise that I should move in the day after the furniture and boxes. In that way, I wouldn't be under the feet of the removal men as they unloaded the lorry, and the bedroom could be made ready well in advance of my homecoming. In turn, I could have a say in the layout and composition of all the other rooms, with no pressure of time or space.

And so it was. I was sorry to be saying goodbye to some of the nurses; many of them had given me such support and encouragement. But as we drove the thirty-odd miles to the new house I was jubilant. I had come such a long way from death's door.

I drove my wheelchair up the little ramp into a hall full of boxes. There was an enormous amount to be done, and although I could do all the thinking, I couldn't help with the physical work. That was to be the way of things from now on. Far from my homecoming being an end – an end to the nightmare, an end to all the difficulties (as I had once hoped) – it was just the beginning.

A new home – our own home. A civilian life – at last. And, something I had never considered – even in my wildest dreams – a new way of life? A life where I couldn't walk, couldn't drive my car. Couldn't work, nor speak properly. A life in which I couldn't clean my own house, dig the garden, or entertain my guests. One where I had to watch while others had free reign in my kitchen. And one in which I couldn't wash myself, feed myself, scratch my nose, or wipe my bum. A challenge?

Back in the early days, soon after it had become obvious that I had survived the stroke, one of the doctors asked me whether survival was worth it.

Time will tell . . .

15. And now . . .

Well, nine years have passed and there is still no sign of a miracle. Nor has stem-cell research come up with anything useful. Iain and I have settled down to a new life – very different from the one we left behind. It certainly isn't the one we envisaged for our middle age.

Some things haven't changed though; Iain is still practising as a popular local GP (albeit a civilian, not an RAF one), and I still run the house (albeit with considerable help – both electronic and human). And we are still together – just! During the writing of this chapter Iain confessed to having an affair. I was/am devastated! My rock, my hero, has feet of clay! I suppose, given the strain that this sort of situation inevitably causes, that I shouldn't be surprised, but I thought we were immune.

Our daughters have continued to give us invaluable support. During the past nine years they have each been through university, qualified at their chosen careers and have left home. They keep in close touch – particularly now that this crisis has arisen. Elinor is a doctor and Elisabeth a vet. Elinor has just spent a year in Australia; she came back early to look after me, after the crisis broke, and to give us both some support. Elisabeth started her job at the end of last year, so she was around while I was hospitalised with septicaemia due to an infected kidney stone. I have cause to be grateful to both of them for their support over the years.

As I have Iain. It has been he who bought and maintained my computer and the software which enables me to do so much (such as internet banking, shopping online, emailing, and typing out lists – I am known for my lists). He bought various pieces of physiotherapy equipment for me to use, and contacted the different agencies I needed to keep in touch with. He has learned to cook and is fiercely independent in the kitchen. For eight years, with rare exceptions, he has put me to bed, fed me my meals, and more. In short, I owe him more than I can describe, and we presented to the world a united front . . .

If there are lessons to be learned from this they would include the need for psychological help to be given to spouses long after the official rehabilitation period, and respite should be taken right from the start – even if it does not seem to be required to avoid carers' 'burn-out'.

Another source of support has been my 'personal assistants'. I have been unbelievably fortunate to have had one of my 'team' (Debra) since the start, and Gill, who helps get me up in the mornings, likewise has been with me since the beginning. I have had a succession of additional PAs over the years – some better than others – and I have a good team at the moment. They do such things as my personal care, meals and exercises. Debra and I cook together and go shopping.

Debra has seen me progress from an inert lump with a twisted face who had to be hoisted everywhere and have her drinks thickened to one who does standing transfers, or if I need to use a hoist I now use a 'Stand-Aid'. My face isn't twisted any more, although the left side pulls tight if I am tense or tired. And I can drink everything unthickened – even water, which was forbidden as it used to make me choke.

I can now go to restaurants – my table-manners have improved sufficiently and I am no longer so self-conscious about being fed when in public – and the theatre. I have even started hosting a charity coffee evening.

But I am still paralysed – the only things that reliably move are my head and my right thumb. My speech is still rubbish. A combination of weak breathing, weak vocal chords and tight facial muscles conspire at best to give me an excruciatingly quiet voice, and at worst to render me incomprehensible. This is probably the most disabling 'difficulty' I have, and because of it most people think that I am 'ga-ga'.

I get around in my electric wheelchair and have control of the radio and TV, some lights and a fan. I can even phone out to some pre-programmed numbers! The physiotherapy and speech therapy input has been stopped, so it is up to my PAs and me – and my daughters – to devise exercises and put them into practice.

My mother puts at the end of each email she sends me 'kbo' – keep buggering on! That is precisely what I have to do . . .

Glossary

Angiogram	X-ray of blood vessels, taken after the injection of radio-opaque dye. In my case to show the blood vessels in the brain.
Arterial line	A fine tube inserted into an artery for constant and accurate monitoring of blood pressure, blood gas levels, etc.
Cannula	A fine tube inserted into an artery or vein.
CVA	Cerebrovascular accident – the posh name for stroke.
Endotracheal tube	(ETT or ET tube) A tube passed via the mouth into the trachea (windpipe), usually used to ventilate unconscious patients, for example during operations.
Gastrostomy	An opening into the stomach made surgically through the abdominal wall for the introduction of food via a tube.
HCA	Health Care Assistant.
High Dependency Unit (HDU)	A halfway house between ITU and the ward.
ICU/ITU	Intensive Care/Therapy Unit.
Intubation	The process of passing an endotracheal tube.
IV infusion	A drip.
Light Writer	A machine producing an electronic voice from words 'typed' (by whatever means) into a computer, e.g. the sort of thing used by Stephen Hawking.

Nasogastric tube	(NGT or NG tube) A tube passed through the nose, down the back of the throat and into the stomach for feeding or drainage.
Nebuliser	A system for humidifying air or oxygen before it is breathed in via ET tube, tracheostomy tube or normally. Used to prevent the airways drying out. Can also be used to introduce nebulised drugs.
Nose	(also Swedish Nose) A device placed over the end of a tracheostomy tube to increase humidity and avoid the airways drying out.
Nystagmus	Involuntary rapid, repetitive flicking of the eyes.
PEG	Percutaneous endoscopic gastrostomy – the usual type of gastrostomy tube, placed using an endoscope passed into the stomach through the mouth.
Tilt table	A hard 'bed' to which the patient is securely strapped with feet on a footplate. An attached motor rotates the 'bed' from the horizontal position to the vertical. Thus, the patient 'stands up' and the body receives some correct orientation.
Tinnitus	Ringing or hissing in the ears.
Tracheostomy	An incision made through the front of the neck into the windpipe to assist breathing.
Tracheostomy tube	Bent tube passed through the tracheostomy to keep it open to allow breathing and suction of the airways.
Urinary catheter	A tube passed into the bladder to drain the urine into a catheter bag. Usually held in place by a balloon.

Urethral catheter	The usual method of placing a urinary catheter – passed into the bladder through the urethra. Usually a temporary arrangement.
Suprapubic catheter	A urinary catheter passed directly into the bladder through a hole made surgically in the abdominal wall. Used for permanent catheterisation.